The Gastric Sleeve Cookbook UK 2022

Carefully Selected, Easy and Delicious Gastric Sleeve Bariatric Recipes for Sustainable Better Health and Keeping the Weight Off for Good. 28 Day Meal Plan & Journal Included

Author: Sarah Roberts

Table of Contents

Benefits And the Latest Scientific Research On The Gastric Sleeve Surgery

Gastric sleeve surgery is traditionally reserved for people who suffer from obesity and have not been able to sustain weight loss in other ways. Also known as bariatric surgery, this is a tool that is designed to help people who are at risk of major health conditions as a result of their weight problems. It can lower the risk of some serious conditions that could become life threatening if not treated promptly.

Weight loss surgery used to be seen as a high risk for gains that were only cosmetic, but this was before we understood the full implications of long-term obesity and the impact that being overweight can have on all the organs. Being obese massively increases the risk of many diseases that could prove fatal, including heart disease and kidney disease.

Losing weight sustainably is an ongoing issue that many people struggle with, especially in today's society. However, bariatric surgery is a possible solution for some of these people, offering long-term control over eating habits and weight loss.

It's thought that approximately 90 per cent of patients who undergo gastric sleeve surgery will lose around half of their body weight and manage to maintain this weight loss in the long term. This can improve mental health as well as physical health, reduce pain, and make it easier for patients to exercise and meet their weight-loss goals consistently.

It's thought that this kind of weight loss can reduce your risk of things like liver cancer and fatty liver disease by as much as 88 per cent. It can also reduce the risk of strokes and cardiovascular issues by around 70 per cent.

You should only consider this kind of surgery if it is being put forward to you by a doctor that you trust. There are some risks associated with gastric sleeve surgery and while it is certainly a good option for some, it is not something that you should undertake lightly or without a solid understanding of the potential drawbacks.

What To Do Before and After The Surgery For A Safe And Easy Procedure

You will be given a specific diet to follow both before and after the surgery, and it's extremely important to stick to this throughout, or you could increase the risks of something going wrong during or after the surgery.

The diet will usually begin two weeks before the surgery is scheduled, and you will find that your calories and carbohydrates are seriously restricted. You may be given a caloric goal, and you will mostly be eating lean proteins and vegetables. You must follow this diet, or discuss with your doctor if you are having any issues that need to be addressed.

You will then be switched onto a clear liquid diet two days before the scheduled surgery. Often, this will include caffeine-free drinks and no-sugar drinks. You will be given advice on what you can consume by your doctor.

This clear liquid diet will usually continue after the procedure for around one or two weeks, and then other foods can gradually be introduced. You will be given a specific plan to follow, and there is more information about this under the heading Explanation Of The Multiple Meal Plan Stages – 4-6 Week Meal Plan.

Staying hydrated is crucial, so if you are having an issue with this, you should consult with your healthcare professional. Sugar must be avoided, as consuming it may cause major adverse reactions, such as vomiting, diarrhoea, and severe nausea. Caffeine and carbonated drinks may also be problematic, and should not be consumed

You may find that you can reintroduce these drinks into your diet later, but they may always cause issues. This is something you should take into consideration when choosing whether to have the surgery.

Recovery times from gastric sleeve surgery can vary, but you should be aware that it will often be up to two months before you can eat normally again. You should use this time to build healthy eating habits that will keep you on track when your menu expands.

Fundamentals Of the Gastric Sleeve Diet – Everything You Need To Know

One of the key aspects of the gastric sleeve diet is to reduce your intake of sugar, which contributes massively to weight gain, and does not make you feel full or satisfied. You will need to reduce the amount of sugar you eat in both the short term and the long term, finding other foods to satisfy you and provide the energy that you need.

Many recipes in this book will include unsweetened versions of foods, so look out for unsweetened milk, protein powder, and other alternatives. You may be able to use fruit sugars when you need a sweetener, although even these will need to be eaten in moderation if you wish to keep your weight low. You may also find that natural sweeteners such as honey help you to maintain the diet without feeling as though you can never eat a "treat" food again.

Eggs, vegetables, and lean protein will be the staples of the diet, and you will need to cut out foods like pasta, potatoes (but not sweet potatoes), and rice, which are all high in carbohydrates. Chicken and fish are often good staples, and you will also depend on vegetables such as cauliflowers, celery, onions, cucumber, beans, and courgettes.

Following a gastric sleeve diet often means opting for the low-fat version of foods, such as low-fat Parmesan, mayonnaise, and Greek yogurt.

Many people find that they are better able to keep their weight low if they have multiple small portions of food in a day, rather than one or two big meals, so make sure you are eating regularly. This will stop you from feeling as hungry in between meals, which can reduce the risk of you makin too much food and therefore eating more than you need. If you find that three meals are not enough, try to eat four, but reduce the portion sizes so that you are not eating more food overall. The idea is simply to space it out so that you don't get hungry in between meals.

Explanation Of the Multiple Meal Plan Stages – 4-6 Week Meal Plan

It will usually be at least four to six weeks after the surgery before you are allowed to eat normally again, and it's important to follow the advice of your healthcare professional during this time to avoid complications. The surgery will have had a big impact on your system, and – as with any operation – you need to make sure you are treating your body in a way that is conducive to healing.

In the first week after the surgery, you'll be following a clear liquid diet that consists of little except Jell-O, sugar-free Popsicles, water, and decaffeinated tea or coffee. You cannot eat much else at this time, unless advised by your doctor. All solid foods will be forbidden.

During the second week after your surgery, you will remain on a clear liquid diet, but your options will usually expand. Clear broths, diluted fruit juices, ice cream, non-fat yogurt, breakfast drinks, and thinned cereal will all be reintroduced. You will still be unable to eat solid foods, and doing so may lead to vomiting and other issues.

In the third week, pureed foods should become an option for you. You will need to eat slowly, however, and chew your food thoroughly. Opt for things like jars of baby food, canned fruit, cottage cheese, plain yogurt, mashed avocado, mashed bananas, and soft scrambled eggs. You should still avoid caffeine and sugar, and keep the foods bland. Eating spicy food may lead to heartburn, so it is important to avoid it for the sake of your own comfort.

In week four, solid foods can slowly be brought back into your diet. You will need to opt for easy-to-digest meals, such as low sugar cereals, fruit, soft vegetables (usually well-cooked), low-fat cheese, and fish. You will need to keep sugar, fat, and fibrous foods off the menu, along with high-carbohydrate foods such as pasta. You can slowly bring caffeine back into your diet at this point, but make sure you are consuming it in moderation.

By week five, you can start gradually introducing other foods. Do so slowly, so you can monitor how your body responds to them, and avoid anything that causes stomach upsets or pain. Do not start eating sugary, high-fat foods, as these will contribute to weight gain, undermining the value of the surgery. Try to choose nutritious foods and avoid anything that triggers your old eating habits. Opt for three regular meals each day, minimise snacking, and keep yourself well hydrated at all times.

Post-Op Serving Sizes for Healthy And Easy Weight Loss

Following your surgery, it's not just important to know what you can eat, but how much of it you can have. You need to be very careful, because your stomach size will have been dramatically reduced, and you'll have to realign your expectations of food to fit with this. If you have been eating large portions previously, this can be particularly challenging, and you should approach portion sizes with care. Ask your healthcare professional if you are in doubt about how much to eat.

In general, for the first six weeks after surgery, you will only be consuming about a quarter of a cup or half a cup of whatever you are eating. This reduces the risk of complications, and allows the staple line to heal without being put under any stress.

Over time, of course, you will need to increase the portion sizes, but they will remain the guide for a surprisingly long time – up to six months after surgery. Talk to your doctor about this in more depth, but you shouldn't be looking to increase your portion sizes for at least a few months. Some people increase after three, but many wait longer than this.

However, as time passes, you will need to eat more, and you will gradually expand your portion to around the size of a cup before a year has passed.

Other people find it easier to measure using their hands. A single portion of fruit or vegetables will be around the size of a closed fist. A serving of meat will be about the size of a deck of cards, or the palm of your hand. For cheese, a piece should be approximately the same size as your thumb.

Snacks should be rare, but if you are eating them, stick to one cupped handful. This should be enough to stave off hunger cravings. In general, it's best to avoid snacks entirely, and to spread your food allowance into small meals if you find that you get hungry in between. However, if you do need to snack, keep the portions small.

3 Common Mistakes People Make After The Surgery

Mistake One: Not Drinking Enough

Hydration is crucial when you've had surgery; water plays so many important roles in the body that you must make sure you are getting enough at all times. However, with how busy life can be, you might struggle to drink enough, and if this happens, you should take steps to remind yourself, such as setting an alarm on your phone or measuring out water in advance.

Water will also help with weight loss because it makes you feel fuller and more energized, and it can reduce the risk of certain health issues and surgical complications. Make sure that you are drinking plenty throughout the day, and make time for water breaks, especially when you have just had the surgery.

If you don't like water, try using a squeeze of fruit juice to flavour it, but try to minimize this. A little splash of lemon may be enough to make the difference. Alternatively, try decaffeinated, unsweetened tea without milk. This may help you to increase your water intake, although it's best to drink plain water where you can.

Tied in with this, another trap that people fall into is drinking carbonated drinks in an attempt to keep themselves hydrated. You should not do this; carbonated drinks almost all contain sugar, but they can also cause discomfort after the surgery. It can be hard to tell the difference between actual pain due to complications and gas pain caused by carbonation. Avoid carbonated drinks if possible.

It's important to note that you are better off not drinking water (or other liquids) at the same time as eating. There are a few reasons for this. Firstly, because your stomach is now small, there may not be room for both food and drink in there, and drinking at the same time as eating could lead to you feeling bloated, or even to vomiting. The liquid may cause the food to swell, leaving your stomach overly full.

Secondly, it's possible for water to wash the food through your stomach more quickly, making it hard to tell when you are full, and more challenging to regulate your food intake. The opposite can also happen; if the water fills your stomach up, you may feel full too soon, and this can lead to malnutrition because you won't be eating enough.

Most people recommend leaving at least thirty minutes after eating before you consume any water. This will give your stomach time to process the food and make space for the liquid. A sip or two to ease a dry mouth should be fine, but do not drink with your meals.

Mistake Two: Drinking Alcohol

Alcohol is not your friend when it comes to weight loss, because it contains calories but no nutrition, so it adds to weight gain without giving your body anything useful. You should avoid alcohol, particularly after you have had the surgery, if you want to keep your weight down.

Furthermore, alcohol could be problematic after the surgery because it will enter your bloodstream much more quickly than before. This makes it easy to get drunk without meaning to, which could be dangerous.

If you wish to reintroduce alcohol after some time has passed, consult your doctor for advice on how to do this. It may be possible, but it is best to have professional advice before you attempt it.

Mistake Three: Not Following Your Diet

The post-op diet can be hard to stick to. It involves long-term commitment and discipline, and it can be a real test of your fortitude – but not following it is a major mistake that can jeopardize your health and recovery.

If you don't stick to the stipulations, especially in the early stages, you are at risk of complications. You need to lose weight at a pre-determined rate and avoid putting stress on your stomach, and this can only be done by following the guidelines you have been given. Do not try to reintroduce solid foods straight away or "cheat" on your diet. It could cause gastrointestinal problems or serious complications.

If you are having problems with the diet, talk to your medical practitioner. They may be able to give you further resources or support to help you through.

Even months or years after the surgery, you will need to be vigilant and disciplined about what you eat. You should not be reintroducing sugar or empty carbohydrates to your diet; you need to eat sensibly and make healthy choices to ensure that you lose weight as intended, and keep it off. The post-op diet will help you on the first steps, but the commitment must be maintained in the long term

Foods You Must Avoid

Although you do have a reasonable amount of choice about the foods you eat, there are certain foods that you must avoid once you have had gastric food surgery, no matter how tempting they are. Here are a few things that should be off your menu for the sake of your stomach and your comfort:

- Tough red meat
- Pretzels
- Rice cakes
- Popcorn
- Pastries
- Alcohol
- Caffeinated drinks
- Dry cereal (add milk and allow it to soak in)
- Rice
- Pasta
- Fibrous fruits and vegetables, including corn (although this should be okay once your stomach has adjusted)
- Bacon
- Whole milk
- Sausage
- Butter
- Sugary fruit juices
- Spicy food
- Potatoes

Every patient's journey is different, so you may find that many of these foods are things you can reintroduce after a while. You will see corn used in the recipes included in this book, because it is a valuable source of nutrients and most people can tolerate it after some time has passed – but it's a good idea to introduce it slowly and cautiously. If you find that your body rejects a certain kind of food the first time you try it, wait for a few weeks before trying it again, and keep the portion very small. This increases the chances of your stomach dealing with it properly.

Some of these foods, such as bacon, pasta, bread, and whole milk, are ones that you may wish to avoid as much as possible, even once your stomach feels better. However, it is still okay to have small amounts of them when you have healed from the surgery; you do not have to cut them out entirely. As long as they are something you eat rarely and you only have small portions, they should not cause any problems.

Approved Food List

You are probably even more interested in what foods you can eat after gastric sleeve surgery, so let' look at those next. As mentioned, however, everyone's recovery experience is different, and you should approach all new foods with care. Do not eat a large piece of something the first time you consume it, or even the first few times. Take small bites, eat slowly, and only introduce one new foo at a time.

This will make it easier to work out if something has upset your stomach. If you introduce five new foods at once and have a bad reaction, you won't know which of the foods set it off, or if it was a combination of having multiple new things to deal with at once. Therefore, whenever you want to add something to your diet, you should eat it on its own, or alongside foods that you already know are safe.

With that said, let's look at the foods that are generally considered safe for those who have had gastric sleeve surgery once they are eating normally again (i.e. not on the clear liquid or puree stage

- Almond butter
- Almond flour
- Apples
- Avocados
- Bananas
- Broccoli
- Chicken
- Salmon
- Beef sirloin
- Cauliflower
- Chickpeas
- Cottage cheese
- Cream cheese

- Cucumbers
- Eggs
- Mayonnaise
- Tomatoes
- Yogurt
- Sweet potatoes
- Spinach
- Mushrooms
- Raspberries
- Mangoes
- Pork
- Leeks
- Onions

- Lemons
- Olives
- Honey
- Cream
- Turkey
- Ginger
- Coconut and cocon products (e.g. butte oil, milk, etc.)
- Blueberries
- Grapes
- Green beans
- Pumpkin

You will find these ingredients and many more included in the following recipes. As long as you are introducing foods slowly and carefully, you can eat most things, but it is important to think about the fat and sugar content of them all. Do not add empty carbohydrates to your meals. Instead, opt for protein-rich and nutritionally dense foods that will give you everything you need to stay healthy without having to eat a lot.

Note that it's a good idea to cook everything you eat after gastric sleeve surgery thoroughly (besides foods that are eaten raw, like fruit). This is particularly true for meats and vegetables, because cooking ensures that they are easy to digest and gentle on your system. Give turkey, chicken, etc., a few more minutes in the pan to ensure that it is truly tender. Steam vegetables for a little longer than usual – and so on. Soft, well-cooked foods are less likely to cause digestive issues.

Approved Snacks

Snacking should be rare after gastric sleeve surgery, but at times, you will just need an energy boost and something to make you feel full, and it's far better to choose healthy snacks than to risk falling into the trap of crisps, sodas, and sugary treats.

If you are going to snack, it's a good idea to portion up your snacks in advance so that you aren't tempted to keep picking at them. For example, if you are going to eat nuts, you can put the amount that you are allowing in small containers, rather than just taking them from the main bag. This is the best way to control your portions and ensure you aren't overdoing it with your snacks.

Some popular and easy snacks that you can try include:

- Cashew nuts
- Pecan nuts
- Strawberries
- Cottage cheese
- Almonds
- Blueberries
- Boiled egg halves
- Hummus

- Peanut butter
- Yogurt
- Cucumbers
- Bell pepper slices
- Melon balls
- Roasted chickpeas
- Guacamole

Remember to limit your snacks to a handful, even if they seem healthy and you don't feel immediately full after eating them. It can sometimes take a little while for the food to "register" with your system, and you will probably find that a small amount will deal with the hunger cravings if you give yourself a bit of time.

Drink plenty of water around your snacks, but not at the same time. This should also help you to feel full and energized throughout the day.

Gastric Sleeve Bariatric Cooking Tips For Easy And Tasty Meals For Sustainable Weight Loss

Tip One: Include Protein

One of the most important things about bariatric cooking is to focus on protein, because this will make you feel fuller and more satisfied, and reduce the risk of overeating. Don't try to make your entire diet consist of vegetables and fruit, because you won't stay healthy or feel satisfied this way. Try to think about the protein component of each meal, and ensure that protein is at the centre of at least some of your meals. You should then think about low-starch vegetables, and build your meal plans based on these two things. This will help you to feel satisfied and get all the nutrients that you need from your diet. Most people should be consuming between sixty and eighty grams of protein every day.

Tip Two: Batch Cook

Wherever possible, it's a good idea to have some suitable meals prepared in advance, because there may be days when you don't feel like cooking, especially in the weeks following your surgery. Tinned soups can be a good option if you really can't cook, but batch cooking is also a great idea. Find meals you like, and make small, controlled portions of these for your freezer. This will help you to eat the correct amount, and ensure you always have something healthy to hand.

Tip Three: Use Your Air Fryer

You'll see that there is an entire section dedicated to air fryer recipes. That's because this is a great way to enjoy some good "treat" foods like drumsticks and burgers without ruining your diet. The air fryer lets you have crispy fried food without the heavy grease and fat usually involved, so it's a great way to make your weight loss sustainable. You can still eat the things you love – but in healthier forms.

Tip Four: Introduce Foods Slowly

As mentioned above, you should add foods back into your diet slowly, even if they have never caused you problems before. If a recipe calls for a couple of foods that you haven't eaten since the surgery, consider omitting one until you know that the other is safe. This can make it easier to stay in control in the kitchen, and avoid upsetting your stomach.

Stage 1: Clear Liquid Recipes

Fruit Juice

Servings|2   Time|10 minutes
Nutritional Content (per serving):
Cal| 401   Fat| 1.6g   Protein| 2.5g   Carbs| 99.6g   Fiber| 15g

Ingredients:

- Large green apples (5, cored and sliced)
- Fresh lime juice (15 milliliters)
- Seedless white grapes (330 grams)

Directions:

1. Add all ingredients into a juicer and extract the juice according to the manufacturer's method.
2. Through a cheesecloth-lined strainer, strain the juice and serve immediately.

Carrot & Lemon Juice

Servings|2   Time|10 minutes
Nutritional Content (per serving):
Cal| 107   Fat| 0.1g   Protein| 2.2g   Carbs| 26g   Fiber| 6.6g

Ingredients:

- Carrots (500 grams, trimmed and scrubbed)
- Water (240 milliliters)
- Lemons (2, peeled and seeded)

Directions:

1. Add all ingredients in a high-power blender and pulse until well combined.
2. Through a cheesecloth-lined strainer, strain the juice and serve immediately.

Lemonade

Servings|8   Time|10 minutes
Nutritional Content (per serving):
Cal| 6   Fat| 0.2g   Protein| 0.2g   Carbs| 0.5g   Fiber| 0.1g

Ingredients:

- ❖ Fresh lemon juice (180 milliliters)
- ❖ Water (1920 milliliters)
- ❖ Lemon stevia drops (5 milliliters)
- ❖ Ice cubes, as required

Directions:

1. In a pitcher, place lemon juice and stevia and stir to combine.
2. Add the water and fill the pitcher with ice before serving.

Citrus Cucumber Sports Drink

Servings|3   Time|10 minutes
Nutritional Content (per serving):
Cal| 19   Fat| 0.2g   Protein| 0.8g   Carbs| 4.8g   Fiber| 0.9g

Ingredients:

- ❖ Lime (1, sliced)
- ❖ Cucumber (1, sliced)
- ❖ Water (1440 milliliters)
- ❖ Lemon (1, sliced)
- ❖ Fresh mint leaves (5 grams)

Directions:

1. In a large glass jar, place fruit, cucumber and mint and pour water on top.
2. Cover the jar with a lid tightly and refrigerate for 2-4 hours before serving.

Simple Coffee

Servings|2   Time|10 minutes
Nutritional Content (per serving):
Cal| 0   Fat| 0g   Protein| 0g   Carbs| 0g   Fiber| 0g

Ingredients:

- ❖ Decaffeinated instant coffee powder (5-10 grams)
- ❖ Liquid stevia (3-4 drops)
- ❖ Boiling water (480 milliliters)

Directions:

1. In 2 mugs, divide coffee, stevia and boiling water and stir to combine.
2. Serve hot.

Simple Black Tea

Servings|2   Time|10 minutes
Nutritional Content (per serving):
Cal| 26   Fat| 0g   Protein| 0g   Carbs| 6.7g   Fiber| 00g

Ingredients:

- ❖ Water (960 milliliters)
- ❖ Maple syrup (20 grams)
- ❖ Black tea leaves (5 grams

Directions:

1. In a medium-sized saucepan, add water and bring to a boil.
2. Stir in the tealeaves and turn off the heat.
3. Immediately, cover the pan and steep for 3 minutes.
4. Add maple syrup and stir until dissolved.
5. Strain the tea in mugs and serve immediately.

Spiced Ginger Tea

Servings|4   Time|25 minutes
Nutritional Content (per serving):
Cal| 29   Fat| 0.1g   Protein| 0.1g   Carbs| 7.3g   Fiber| 0.2g

Ingredients:

- Water (1440 milliliters)
- Fresh ginger (1 (2½-centimeter) piece, chopped)
- Pinch of ground cinnamon
- Lemon (½, seeded and sliced)
- Maple syrup (40 grams)
- Pinch of ground turmeric

Directions:

1. In a saucepan, add all ingredients over medium-high heat and bring to a boil.
2. Adjust the heat to medium-low and simmer for about 10-12 minutes.
3. Strain into cups and serve hot.

Chicken Broth

Servings|12   Time|5½ hours
Nutritional Content (per serving):
Cal| 357   Fat| 12.6g   Protein| 45.1g   Carbs| 14g   Fiber| 3.7g

Ingredients:

- Olive oil (15 milliliters)
- Carrots (455 grams, peeled and chopped)
- Turnip (455 grams, peeled and chopped)
- Water (3 liters)
- Fresh dill bunch (1)
- Fresh parsley bunch (1)
- Medium onion (1, chopped)
- Celery stalks (4, chopped)
- Parsnip (455 grams, peeled and chopped)
- Whole chicken (1 (1820-gram, gizzards removed)
- Ground black pepper, as required

Directions:

1. Heat olive oil in a large-sized soup pan over medium heat and sauté onion, carrots and celery for about 5 minutes.
2. Add the parsnips and turnips and sauté for about 5 minutes.
3. Add the chicken, water, herbs and black pepper and bring to a boil.
4. Adjust the heat to low and simmer for about 4-5 hours, skimming the foam from the surface occasionally.
5. Through a fine-mesh sieve, strain the broth and serve hot.

Lemon Gelatin

Servings|8   Time|15 minutes
Nutritional Content (per serving):
Cal| 348   Fat| 1.3g   Protein| 2.4g   Carbs| 90.6g   Fiber| 14g

Ingredients:

- Grass-fed gelatin powder (30 grams)
- Boiling water (360 milliliters)
- Stevia extract (10 milliliters)
- Cold water (720 milliliters, divided)
- Fresh lemon juice (270 milliliters)

Directions:

1. In a bowl, soak the gelatin in 360 milliliters of cold water. Set aside for about 5 minutes.
2. After 5 minutes, add the boiling water and stir until gelatin dissolves.
3. Add the remaining cold water, lemon juice and stevia extract and stir until dissolved completely.
4. Divide the mixture into 2 baking dishes and refrigerate until set before serving.

Kiwi & Cucumber Popsicles

Servings|8   Time|15 minutes
Nutritional Content (per serving):
Cal| 60   Fat| 0.3g   Protein| 1g   Carbs| 14.5g   Fiber| 1.8g

Ingredients:

- Cucumbers (455 grams, chopped)
- Fresh lime juice (120 milliliters)
- Water (200 milliliters)
- Kiwis (4, peeled)
- Fresh mint leaves (40 grams)
- Maple syrup (75 grams)

Directions:

1. Add all ingredients in a high-power blender and pulse until smooth.
2. Transfer the mixture into the popsicle molds and freeze for 4 hours before serving.

Stage 2: Pureed Food Recipes

Vanilla Smoothie

Servings|2 Time|10 minutes
Nutritional Content (per serving):
Cal| 160   Fat| 4.4g   Protein| 26.4g   Carbs| 2g   Fiber| 0.9g

Ingredients:

- Unsweetened protein powder (60 grams)
- Organic vanilla extract (5 milliliters)
- Ice cubes (4-6)
- Almond butter (15 grams)
- Unsweetened almond milk (360 milliliters)
- Liquid stevia (6-8 drops)

Directions:

1. In a high-power blender, add all the ingredients and pulse until smooth.
2. Pour the smoothie into 2 serving glasses and serve immediately.

Egg Salad

Servings|2 Time|10 minutes
Nutritional Content (per serving):
Cal| 99   Fat| 7g   Protein| 6.2g   Carbs| 2.8g   Fiber| 0g

Ingredients:

- Hard-boiled eggs (2, peeled and sliced)
- Ground black pepper, as required
- Plain Low-fat Greek yogurt (20 grams)
- Low-fat mayonnaise (15 grams)

Directions:

1. Place the egg slices in a food processor and pulse until finely chopped.
2. Add the remaining ingredients and pulse until smooth.

Citrus Ricotta

Servings|3   Time|10 minutes
Nutritional Content (per serving):
Cal| 200   Fat| 11.2g   Protein| 16.2g   Carbs| 7.7g   Fiber| 0.2g

Ingredients:

- Low-fat ricotta cheese (1 (425-gram) container)
- Organic vanilla extract (5 milliliters)
- Lime zest (5 grams, grated)
- Lemon extract (5 milliliters)
- Liquid stevia (3-6 drops)

Directions:

1. Add all ingredients in a clean food processor and pulse until smooth.
2. Serve immediately.

Ranch Cottage Cheese

Servings|2   Time|10 minutes
Nutritional Content (per serving):
Cal| 53   Fat| 1.1g   Protein| 8g   Carbs| 2.3g   Fiber| 0g

Ingredients:

- Low-fat cottage cheese with chives (115 grams)
- Pinch of ground black pepper
- Dry ranch dressing mix (5½ grams)

Directions:

1. In a medium-sized serving bowl, add all ingredients and stir to combine.
2. Serve immediately.

White Beans Puree

Servings|2   Time|10 minutes
Nutritional Content (per serving):
Cal| 74   Fat| 0.7g   Protein| 5g   Carbs| 11.9g   Fiber| 4.8g

Ingredients:

- Canned white beans (90 grams, rinsed)
- Low-fat chicken broth (120 milliliters)
- Fresh lemon juice (15 milliliters)
- Jarred jalapeño juice (10 milliliters)

Directions:

1. Place the black beans, lemon juice and juice from jarred jalapeños in a small saucepan over medium heat and stir to combine.
2. Place the saucepan of beans mixture over medium heat and cook for about 3-5 minutes, stirring frequently.
3. Stir in the chicken broth and remove from heat.
4. In a blender, add the beans mixture and pulse until smooth.
5. Transfer the mixture into a serving bowl and set aside to cool slightly.
6. In the bowl of beans puree, add the protein powder and stir until well combined.
7. Serve immediately.

Chicken Liver Pâté

Servings|4   Time|28 minutes
Nutritional Content (per serving):
Cal| 181   Fat| 9.4g   Protein| 17.1g   Carbs| 7.8g   Fiber| 1.4g

Ingredients:

- Low-fat spread (15 grams)
- Chicken livers (225 grams)
- Pinch of salt
- Ground black pepper, as required
- Low-fat butter (45 grams, melted)
- Red onion (1, finely chopped
- Garlic clove (1, crushed)
- Concentrated tomato puree (15 grams)
- Fat-free fromage frais (35-40 grams)

Directions:

1. In a non-stick frying pan, melt the spread over medium-low heat and sauté the onion and garlic for about 5 minutes.
2. Add in chicken livers and cook for about 5-8 minutes or until cooked through.
3. Stir in the tomato puree, salt and black pepper and remove from heat. Set aside to cool.
4. Place the chicken liver mixture and fromage frais into a food processor and pulse until smooth.
5. Transfer the mixture into to a serving bowl.
6. With a plastic wrap, cover the dish and refrigerate for 2 hours before serving.

Chicken Puree

Servings|2   Time|10½ minutes
Nutritional Content (per serving):
Cal| 53   Fat| 1.5g   Protein| 7.7g   Carbs| 2.1g   Fiber| 0.5g

Ingredients:

- Canned chicken (85 milliliters)
- Italian seasoning (5 grams)
- Ground black pepper (1 gram)
- Tomato sauce (55 grams)
- Salt (1 gram)

Directions:

1. Place all ingredients in a small-sized blender and pulse until smooth.
2. Transfer the mixture into a microwave-safe bowl and microwave for about 30 seconds.
3. Serve immediately.

Tuna Puree

Servings|4   Time|10 minutes
Nutritional Content (per serving):
Cal| 82   Fat| 2.9g   Protein| 10g   Carbs| 3.8g   Fiber| 0g

Ingredients:

- Water-packed tuna (1 (150-gram) can, drained)
- Fat-free plain Greek yogurt (35 grams)
- Relish (15 grams)
- Low-fat mayonnaise (30 grams)
- Ground black pepper, as required

Directions:

1. Add all ingredients in a clean food processor and pulse until smooth.
2. Serve immediately.

Smoked Salmon Pâté

Servings|2   Time|10 minutes
Nutritional Content (per serving):
Cal| 103   Fat| 3.1g   Protein| 14.1g   Carbs| 4.5g   Fiber| 0.5g

Ingredients:

- Fresh smoked salmon (130 grams)
- Dried dill weed (5 grams)
- Salt (1 gram)
- Ground black pepper (1 gram)
- Fat-free plain Greek yogurt (70 grams)
- Fresh lemon juice (20 milliliters

Directions:

1. Add all ingredients in a clean food processor and pulse until smooth.
2. Serve immediately.

Shrimp Puree

Servings|8   Time|10 minutes
Nutritional Content (per serving):
Cal| 177   Fat| 10.5g   Protein| 15.2g   Carbs| 5.4g   Fiber| 0.3g

Ingredients:

- Low-fat cream cheese (225 grams, softened)
- Sugar-free cocktail sauce (225 grams)
- Cooked shrimp (455 grams)
- Fat-free plain Greek yogurt (140 grams)

Directions:

1. Add all ingredients in a clean food processor and pulse until smooth.
2. Serve immediately.

Stage 3: Soft Food Recipes

Banana Smoothie

Servings|2   Time|10 minutes
Nutritional Content (per serving):
Cal| 306   Fat| 4.3g   Protein| 19.7g   Carbs| 51.3g   Fiber| 6.4g

Ingredients:

- ❖ Gluten-free rolled oats (50 grams)
- ❖ Bananas (2, peeled and sliced)
- ❖ Ground cinnamon (1¼ grams)
- ❖ Fat-free plain Greek yogurt (280 grams)
- ❖ Unsweetened almond milk (240 milliliters)

Directions:

1. In a high-power blender, add all the ingredients and pulse until smooth.
2. Pour the smoothie into 2 serving glasses and serve immediately.

Raspberry Smoothie Bowl

Servings|2   Time|10 minutes
Nutritional Content (per serving):
Cal| 192   Fat| 1.5g   Protein| 10.4g   Carbs| 36.5g   Fiber| 6g

Ingredients:

- ❖ Frozen raspberries (260 grams)
- ❖ Unsweetened whey protein powder (10 grams)
- ❖ Unsweetened almond milk (120 milliliters)
- ❖ Fat-free plain yogurt (70 grams

Directions:

1. In a blender, add frozen strawberries and pulse for about 1 minute.
2. Add the almond milk, yogurt and protein powder and pulse until smooth.
3. Transfer the smoothie mixture into 2 serving bowls evenly and with your favorite topping.

Veggie Smoothie Bowl

Servings|2   Time|10 minutes
Nutritional Content (per serving):
Cal| 126   Fat| 7.7g   Protein| 6.4g   Carbs| 9.1g   Fiber| 5g

Ingredients:

- Courgette (125 grams, chopped roughly)
- Cauliflower florets (50 grams, chopped roughly)
- Hemp hearts (20 grams)
- Ground cinnamon (5 grams)
- Liquid stevia (2-3 drops)
- Frozen spinach leaves (50 grams)
- Unsweetened almond milk (240 milliliters)
- Almond butter (30 grams)
- Organic vanilla extract (5 milliliters)

Directions:

1. In a high-power blender, put all the ingredients and pulse until smooth.
2. Transfer into 2 serving bowls and serve with your favorite topping.

Eggs & Cheddar Scramble

Servings|6 Time|18 minutes
Nutritional Content (per serving):
Cal| 226   Fat| 17.6g   Protein| 16g   Carbs| 2.5g   Fiber| 16g

Ingredients:

- Olive oil (30 milliliters)
- Eggs (12, beaten lightly)
- Low-fat cheddar cheese (115 grams, shredded)
- Small onion (1, finely chopped)
- Ground black pepper, as required

Directions:

1. In a large-sized wok, heat oil over medium heat and sauté the onion for about 4-5 minutes.
2. Add the eggs and black pepper and cook for about 3 minutes, stirring continuously.
3. Stir in the cheese and serve immediately.

Egg & Avocado Salad

Servings|4   Time|15 minutes
Nutritional Content (per serving):
Cal| 248   Fat| 20.5g   Protein| 10g   Carbs| 8.4g   Fiber| 5.3g

Ingredients:

- Hard-boiled eggs (6, peeled)
- Fresh lemon juice (15 milliliters)
- Onion (60 grams, chopped)
- Salt (1½ grams)
- Ripe avocados (2, peeled and pitted)
- Celery stalks (2, chopped)
- Dijon mustard (5 grams)
- Pinch of ground black pepper

Directions:

1. Cut each boiled egg in half and transfer the yolks into a small-sized bowl.
2. Cut the whites into small pieces and transfer into another bowl.
3. In the bowl of egg yolks, add 1 avocado and with a fork, mash until well combined.
4. Add the mustard, lemon juice, black pepper and mix well. Set aside.
5. Chop the remaining avocado and transfer into the bowl of egg whites.
6. Add the celery and onion whites and mix well.
7. Add the egg yolk mixture and gently stir to combine.
8. Refrigerate to chill for about 2 hours before serving.

Tuna Stuffed Avocado

Servings|2   Time|15 minutes
Nutritional Content (per serving):
Cal| 302   Fat| 20.3g   Protein| 20.6g   Carbs| 11.9g   Fiber| 7.2g

Ingredients:

- ❖ Canned water-packed tuna (115 grams, drained and flaked)
- ❖ Avocado (1, halved and pitted)
- ❖ Fat-free plain Greek yogurt (70 grams)
- ❖ Pinch of cayenne pepper
- ❖ Fresh lime juice (15 milliliters)
- ❖ Onion (30 grams, finely chopped)
- ❖ Dijon mustard (5 grams)
- ❖ Ground black pepper, as required

Directions:

1. With a small-sized spoon, scoop out the flesh from the middle of each avocado half and transfer into a bowl.
2. Add the lime juice and mash until well combined.
3. Add remaining ingredients and stir to combine.
4. Divide the chicken mixture in avocado halves evenly and serve immediately.

Creamy Cauliflower Bake

Servings|3   Time|20 minutes
Nutritional Content (per serving):
Cal| 170   Fat| 13.8g   Protein| 6g   Carbs| 5.8g   Fiber| 2.2g

Ingredients:

- ❖ Cauliflower head (1, florets removed and chopped)
- ❖ Ground black pepper, as required
- ❖ Heavy cream (60 grams)
- ❖ Low-fat butter (15 grams)
- ❖ Low-fat cheddar cheese (45 grams, shredded)

Directions:

1. Preheat your oven to broiler. Lightly grease 3 ramekins.
2. In a saucepan of boiling water, cook cauliflower for about 4-5 minutes.
3. Through a colander, drain the cauliflower well.
4. In a bowl, place the cauliflower, and with an immersion blender, blend until pureed.
5. Add the heavy cream, butter and black pepper and mix well.
6. Divide the cauliflower mixture into the prepared ramekins evenly and top each with cheddar cheese.
7. Arrange the ramekins onto a baking sheet.
8. Transfer the baking sheet of ramekins into the oven and broil for about 3-5 minutes or until cheese is bubbly.
9. Serve warm.

Cheesy Marinara Bake

Servings|5   Time|30 minutes
Nutritional Content (per serving):
Cal| 168   Fat| 10.1g   Protein| 13.4g   Carbs| 5.7g   Fiber| 0.3g

Ingredients:

- Part-skim ricotta cheese (425 grams)
- Dried basil (1 gram)
- Ground black pepper, as required
- Low-fat Parmesan cheese (85 grams, grated)
- Garlic powder (1 gram)
- Sugar-free marinara sauce (95 grams)

Directions:

1. Preheat your oven to 180 degrees C.
2. Grease 5 ramekins.
3. Arrange the ramekins onto a baking sheet.
4. In a large-sized bowl, add ricotta, Parmesan, basil, garlic powder and black pepper and mix well.
5. Divide the cheese mixture into the prepared ramekins evenly and top each with marinara sauce.
6. Arrange the ramekins onto a baking sheet.
7. Bake for approximately 20 minutes.
8. Serve warm.

Tomato Soup

Servings|4   Time|30 minutes
Nutritional Content (per serving):
Cal| 90   Fat| 7.4g   Protein| 1.2g   Carbs| 6.5g   Fiber| 1.9g

Ingredients:

- Olive oil (30 milliliters)
- Tomatoes (350 grams, finely chopped)
- Pinch of salt
- ground black pepper, as required
- Onion, chopped (120 grams)
- Dried thyme (1½ grams)
- Fresh basil leaves (10 grams, chopped)
- Water (720 milliliters)

Directions:

1. In a large-sized soup pan, heat oil over medium heat and sauté onion for about 4-5 minutes.
2. Add the tomatoes, thyme and water and bring to a boil.
3. Now adjust the heat to low and simmer, covered for about 15 minutes.
4. Remove the soup pan from heat and set aside to cool slightly.
5. In a blender, add soup in batches and pulse until smooth.
6. Return the soup in the same pan over medium heat.
7. Stir in basil and cook for about 3-4 minutes.
8. Season with salt and black pepper and serve hot.

Courgette Soup

Servings|6   Time|45 minutes
Nutritional Content (per serving):
Cal| 104   Fat| 6g   Protein| 5.4g   Carbs| 8.5g   Fiber| 2.1g

Ingredients:

- ❖ Olive oil (30 milliliters)
- ❖ Garlic cloves (6, minced)
- ❖ Fresh thyme sprigs (2)
- ❖ Low-fat vegetable broth (960 milliliters)
- ❖ Fresh lemon juice (30 milliliters)
- ❖ Small onions (2, chopped)
- ❖ Courgette (800 grams, cubed)
- ❖ Fresh rosemary sprigs (2)
- ❖ Cayenne pepper (1¼ grams)
- ❖ Ground black pepper, as required

Directions:

1. In a large-sized soup pan, heat oil over medium heat and sauté the onions for about 5-6 minutes.
2. Add in garlic and sauté for about 45-60 seconds.
3. Add the courgette and cook for about 5 minutes, stirring occasionally.
4. Stir in the thyme, rosemary, broth, cayenne pepper and black pepper and bring to a boil.
5. Now adjust the heat to low and cook, covered for about 15-20 minutes.
6. Remove from heat and discard the herb sprigs.
7. Set the pan aside to cool slightly.
8. In a large blender, add the soup in 2 batches and pulse until smooth.
9. Return the soup into the same pan over medium heat.
10. Stir in the lemon juice and cook for about 2-3 minutes or until heated completely.
11. Serve hot.

Stage 4: Recipes for Life
Breakfast Recipes

Yogurt & Cheese Bowl

Servings|2 Time|10 minutes
Nutritional Content (per serving):
Cal| 251   Fat| 6.1g   Protein| 13.4g   Carbs| 39.4g   Fiber| 7g

Ingredients:

- Fat-free plain Greek yogurt (140 grams)
- Extra-virgin olive oil (10 milliliters)
- Fresh mixed berries (50 grams)
- Low-fat cottage cheese (75 grams)
- Ground cinnamon (1¼ grams)
- Medium apples (2, cored and cubed)

Directions:

1. In a large-sized bowl, add the yogurt, cheese, oil and cinnamon and mix until well combined.
2. Gently, fold in the apple and berries.
3. Divide the yogurt mixture in 2 serving bowls and serve immediately.

Strawberry Chia Pudding

Servings|4   Time|10 minutes
Nutritional Content (per serving):
Cal| 135   Fat| 7.4g   Protein| 4.8g   Carbs| 30g   Fiber| 9g

Ingredients:

- Unsweetened almond milk (155 milliliters)
- Large soft dates (5, pitted and chopped)
- Fresh strawberries (250 grams)
- Frozen banana (½, peeled and sliced)
- Chia seeds (80 grams)

Directions:

1. Add all ingredients in a clean food processor except for chia seeds and pulse until smooth.
2. Transfer the mixture into a bowl.
3. Add chia seeds and stir to combine well.
4. Refrigerate for 30 minutes, stirring after every 5 minutes.

Banana Porridge

Servings|4   Time|10 minutes
Nutritional Content (per serving):
Cal| 195   Fat| 7.2g   Protein| 3.9g   Carbs| 29.4g   Fiber| 3.9g

Ingredients:

- Large bananas (4, peeled and mashed)
- Ground cinnamon (2½ grams)
- Almond butter (15 grams, softened)
- Fresh blueberries (100 grams)

Directions:

1. In a large-sized bowl, add bananas, almond butter and cinnamon and stir to combine.
2. Top with blueberries and serve.

Overnight Oatmeal

Servings|2   Time|10 minutes
Nutritional Content (per serving):
Cal| 300   Fat| 7.3g   Protein| 9.6g   Carbs| 54.6g   Fiber| 9.7g

Ingredients:

- Gluten-free rolled oats (100 grams)
- Chia seeds (10 grams)
- Fresh blueberries (50 grams)
- Large banana (1, peeled and mashed)
- Unsweetened almond milk (240 milliliters)

Directions:

1. Add all ingredients except for blueberries in a large-sized bowl and mix until well combined.
2. Refrigerate, covered overnight.
3. Serve with the topping of blueberries.

Apple Porridge

Servings|4   Time|15 minutes
Nutritional Content (per serving):
Cal| 180   Fat| 11.1g   Protein| 4.5g   Carbs| 18.9g   Fiber| 4.5g

Ingredients:

- Unsweetened almond milk (480 milliliters)
- Large apples (2, peeled, cored and grated)
- Small apple (½, cored and sliced)
- Walnuts (40 grams, chopped)
- Sunflower seeds (25 grams)
- Organic vanilla extract (5 milliliters)
- Pinch of ground cinnamon

Directions:

1. In a large-sized saucepan, blend together the milk, walnuts, sunflower seeds, grated apple, vanilla and cinnamon over medium-low heat and cook for about 3-5 minutes.
2. Remove from heat and serve with the topping apple slices.

Savory Crepes

Servings|8   Time|23 minutes
Nutritional Content (per serving):
Cal| 51   Fat| 0.9g   Protein| 2.7g   Carbs| 8.4g   Fiber| 2.4g

Ingredients:

- Chickpea flour (105 grams)
- Red chili powder (1 gram)
- Fresh ginger (2½ grams, grated)
- Fresh coriander leaves (10 grams, chopped)
- Green chili (1, seeded and minced)
- Pinch of salt
- Ground black pepper, as required
- Fresh parsley leaves (10 grams, chopped)
- Water (240 milliliters)
- Olive oil cooking spray

Directions:

1. In a large-sized bowl, add flour, salt, chili powder and black pepper and mix well.
2. Add the ginger, coriander and green chili and mix until well combined.
3. Add the water and mix until a smooth mixture forms.
4. Cover the bowl and set aside for about ½-2 hours.
5. Lightly grease a large non-stick wok with cooking spray and heat over medium-high heat.
6. Add the desired amount of mixture and tilt the pan to spread in an even and thin layer.
7. Cook for about 15-20 seconds or until bottom becomes golden brown.
8. Carefully flip the side and cook for about 15-20 seconds more or until golden brown.
9. Repeat with the remaining mixture.
10. Serve warm.

Oatmeal Pancakes

Servings|3   Time|25 minutes
Nutritional Content (per serving):
Cal| 199   Fat| 2.9g   Protein| 5.5g   Carbs| 40g   Fiber| 5g

Ingredients:

- Gluten-free rolled oats (100 grams)
- Unsweetened almond milk (60-120 milliliters)
- Apple cider vinegar (15 milliliters)
- Fresh blueberries (50 grams)
- Medium banana (1, peeled and mashed)
- Organic baking powder (10 grams)
- Maple syrup (20 grams)
- Organic vanilla extract (5 milliliters)

Directions:

1. Add all the ingredients except for blueberries in a large-sized bowl and mix until well combined.
2. Gently fold in the blueberries.
3. Set the pancake mixture aside for about 5-10 minutes.
4. Preheat a large non-stick wok over medium-low heat.
5. Add desired amount of the mixture and spread in an even layer.
6. Immediately cover the wok and cook for about 2-3 minutes or until golden.
7. Carefully flip the pancake and cook for about 1-2 minutes more.
8. Repeat with the remaining mixture.
9. Serve warm.

Oats & Cheese Waffles

Servings|4   Time|26 minutes
Nutritional Content (per serving):
Cal| 348   Fat| 11.3g   Protein| 24g   Carbs| 43g   Fiber| 4g

Ingredients:

- ❖ Gluten-free old-fashioned oats (200 grams)
- ❖ Large eggs (6)
- ❖ Maple syrup (40 grams)
- ❖ Low-fat cottage cheese (320 grams)
- ❖ Organic vanilla extract (2½ milliliters)

Directions:

1. Preheat your waffle iron and then grease it.
2. In a food processor, add the oats, cottage cheese, eggs and vanilla extract and pulse until smooth.
3. Add ¼ of the mixture in the preheated waffle iron and cook for about 3-4 minutes or until waffles become golden brown.
4. Repeat with the remaining mixture.
5. Serve warm with the drizzling of maple syrup.

Beans & Egg Scramble

Servings|2   Time|25 minutes
Nutritional Content (per serving):
Cal| 163   Fat| 9.6g   Protein| 9g   Carbs| 10.9g   Fiber| 2.7g

Ingredients:

- Olive oil (15 milliliters)
- Shallot (1, sliced thinly)
- Pinch of salt
- Ground black pepper, as required
- Canned cannellini beans (145 grams, rinsed and drained)
- Eggs (2, lightly beaten)
- Fresh parsley (5 grams, chopped)

Directions:

1. In a non-stick sauté pan, heat oil over low heat and cook the beans and shallot for about 10 minutes, stirring occasionally.
2. Add the eggs, salt and black pepper and cook for about 3-5 minutes or until done completely, stirring continuously.
3. Remove the scramble from heat and serve immediately with the garnishing of parsley.

Apple Omelet

Servings|2   Time|20 minutes
Nutritional Content (per serving):
Cal| 292   Fat| 19.7g   Protein| 13g   Carbs| 18.3g   Fiber| 2.1g

Ingredients:

- Extra-virgin olive oil (20 milliliters, divided)
- Ground cinnamon (1¼ grams)
- Pinch of ground nutmeg
- Large eggs (4)
- Small green apples (2, cored and sliced thinly)
- Pinch of ground cloves
- Organic vanilla extract (1¼ milliliters)

Directions:

1. In a medium-sized non-stick wok, heat 5 milliliters of oil over medium-low heat.
2. Add apple slices and sprinkle with spices.
3. Cook for about 4-5 minutes, flipping once halfway through.
4. Meanwhile, in a bowl, add the eggs and vanilla extract and beat until fluffy.
5. In the same wok, heat remaining 15 milliliters of oil over medium-low heat.
6. Place the egg mixture over apple slices evenly and cook for about 3-5 minutes or until desired doneness.
7. Carefully turn the pan over a serving plate and serve immediately.

Courgette Frittata

Servings|6   Time|35 minutes
Nutritional Content (per serving):
Cal| 158   Fat| 11.7g   Protein| 11g   Carbs| 3.1g   Fiber| 0.8g

Ingredients:

- Unsweetened almond milk (30 milliliters)
- Olive oil (15 milliliters)
- Garlic clove (1, minced)
- Goat cheese (55 grams, crumbled)
- Eggs (8)
- Ground black pepper, as required
- Medium courgettes (2, cut into ¼-inch thick round slices)

Directions:

1. Preheat your oven to 180 degrees C.
2. In a bowl, add almond milk, eggs and black pepper and black pepper and beat well.
3. In an ovenproof wok, heat oil over medium heat and sauté the garlic for about 1 minute.
4. Stir in the courgette and cook for about 5 minutes.
5. Add the egg mixture and stir for about 1 minute.
6. Sprinkle the cheese on top and immediately transfer the wok into the oven.
7. Bake for approximately 12 minutes or until eggs become set.
   Remove the wok of frittata from oven and set aside to cool for about 5 minutes. Cut into desired-sized wedges and serve.

Green Veggie Quiche

Servings|4   Time|35 minutes
Nutritional Content (per serving):
Cal| 120   Fat| 7g   Protein| 10.2g   Carbs| 4.8g   Fiber| 0.8g

Ingredients:

- Eggs (6)
- Pinch of salt
- Ground black pepper, as required
- Green capsicum (75 grams, seeded and chopped)
- Fresh chives (5 grams, minced)
- Low-fat milk (120 milliliters)
- Fresh baby spinach (60 grams, chopped)
- Green onions (1, chopped)
- Fresh parsley (10 grams, chopped)

Directions:

1. Preheat your oven to 200 degrees C.
2. Lightly grease a pie dish.
3. In a bowl, add eggs, almond milk, salt and black pepper and beat until well combined. Set aside.
4. In another bowl, add the vegetables and herbs and mix well.
5. In the bottom of the prepared pie dish, place the veggie mixture evenly and top with the egg mixture.
6. Bake for approximately 19-20 minutes or until a wooden skewer inserted in the center comes out clean.
7. Remove pie dish from the oven and set aside for about 5 minutes before slicing.
8. Cut the quiche into desired-sized wedges and serve warm.

Spinach & Eggs Bake

Servings|2   Time|32 minutes
Nutritional Content (per serving):
Cal| 161   Fat| 10.2g   Protein| 14.4g   Carbs| 4.3g   Fiber| 2.1g

Ingredients:

- Fresh baby spinach (180 grams)
- Eggs (4)
- Feta cheese (10-15 grams, crumbled)
- Water (30-45 milliliters)
- Ground black pepper, as required
- Fresh chives (5 grams, minced)

Directions:

1. Preheat your oven to 200 degrees C.
2. Lightly grease 2 small baking dishes.
3. In a medium-sized wok, add the spinach and water over medium heat and cook for about 3-4 minutes, stirring occasionally.
4. Remove the wok of spinach from heat and drain the excess water completely.
5. Divide the spinach into prepared baking dishes evenly.
6. Carefully crack 2 eggs in each baking dish over spinach.
7. Sprinkle with black pepper and top with feta cheese evenly.
8. Arrange the baking dishes onto a large cookie sheet.
9. Bake for approximately 15-18 minutes or until desired doneness of eggs.
10. Serve hot with the garnishing of chives.

Chicken & Sweet Potato Hash

Servings|8   Time|50 minutes
Nutritional Content (per serving):
Cal| 197   Fat| 6.8g   Protein| 20.4g   Carbs| 13.8g   Fiber| 2.5g

Ingredients:

- Olive oil (30 milliliters, divided)
- Medium onion (1, chopped)
- Celery stalks (2, chopped)
- Dried thyme (5 grams)
- Large sweet potatoes (2, peeled and cubed)
- Green onions (100 grams, chopped)
- Skinless, boneless chicken breasts (680 grams, cubed)
- Garlic cloves (4, minced)
- Dried thyme (5 grams)
- Fresh lime juice (30 milliliters)
- Ground black pepper, as required

Directions:

1. In a large non-stick wok, heat 15 milliliters of the oil over medium heat and cook the chicken cubes for about 4-5 minutes.
2. With a slotted spoon, transfer the chicken into a bowl.
3. In the same wok, heat the remaining oil over medium heat and sauté the onion and celery for about 3-4 minutes.
4. Add the garlic and thyme and sauté for about 1 minute.
5. Add the sweet potato and cook for about 8-10 minutes.
6. Add the broth and cook for about 8-10 minutes.
7. Add the cooked chicken, lime juice and Green onions and cook for about 5 minutes.
8. Season with black pepper and serve hot.

Blueberry Muffins

Servings|5   Time|27 minutes
Nutritional Content (per serving):
Cal| 137   Fat| 6.5g   Protein| 3.9g   Carbs| 12.4g   Fiber| 3.5g

Ingredients:

- Gluten-free rolled oats (50 grams)
- Flaxseeds (20 grams)
- Pinch of ground nutmeg
- Almond butter (60 grams, softened)
- Organic vanilla extract (2½ milliliters)
- Almond flour (25 grams)
- Baking soda (3 grams)
- Ground cinnamon (2½ grams)
- Egg (1)
- Banana (30-35 grams, peeled and sliced)
- Fresh blueberries (50 grams)

Directions:

1. Preheat your oven to 190 degrees C.
2. Grease 10 cups of a muffin tin.
3. Add all ingredients except for the blueberries in a high-power blender and pulse until smooth and creamy.
4. Transfer the oats mixture into a bowl and gently, fold in blueberries.
5. Transfer the mixture into prepared muffin cups evenly.
6. Transfer the muffin tin into the preheated oven and bake for approximately 11-12 minutes.
7. Remove the muffin tin from oven and place onto a wire rack to cool for about 10 minutes.
8. Carefully invert the muffins onto the wire rack to cool completely before serving.

Lunch Recipes

Berries & Spinach Salad

Servings|4   Time|15 minutes
Nutritional Content (per serving):
Cal| 123   Fat| 8.4g   Protein| 3.3g   Carbs| 11.2g   Fiber| 3g

Ingredients:

For Salad

- Fresh strawberries (125 grams, hulled and sliced)
- Fresh blueberries (190 grams)
- Fresh baby spinach (120 grams)
- Walnuts (30 grams, toasted and chopped)
- Pinch of salt

For Dressing

- Balsamic vinegar (15 milliliters)
- Fresh lime juice (15 milliliters)
- Olive oil ((15 milliliters)
- Liquid stevia (2-3 drops)
- Ground black pepper, as required

Directions:

1. For salad: in a large serving bowl, add the strawberries and spinach and mix.
2. For dressing: in a small bowl, add all the ingredients and beat until well combined.
3. Place the dressing over salad and toss to coat well.
4. Top with walnuts and serve immediately.

Cucumber & Tomato Salad

Servings|5   Time|10 minutes
Nutritional Content (per serving):
Cal| 73   Fat| 5.9g   Protein| 1.1g   Carbs| 5.4g   Fiber| 1.3g

Ingredients:

- Cucumbers (300 grams, peeled and chopped)
- Extra-virgin olive oil (30 milliliters)
- Tomatoes (400 grams, peeled and chopped)
- Fresh lime juice (30 milliliters)
- Salt, as required

Directions:

1. In a large-sized salad bowl, add all ingredients and toss to coat well.
2. Serve immediately.

Turkey & Beans Lettuce Wraps

Servings|2 Time|28 minutes
Nutritional Content (per serving):
Cal| 244   Fat| 15.2g   Protein| 15g   Carbs| 13.9g   Fiber| 5.3g

Ingredients:

- Lean ground turkey (115 grams)
- Sugar-free tomato sauce (35 grams)
- Ground black pepper, as required
- Tomato (200 grams, chopped)
- Fresh coriander (5 grams, chopped)
- Onion (30 grams, minced)
- Ground cumin (1 gram)
- Extra-virgin olive oil (15 milliliters
- Cooked black beans (35 grams)
- Small avocado (½, peeled, pitted and chopped)
- Large lettuce leaves (4)

Directions:

1. In a bowl, add the turkey, onion, tomato sauce, cumin and black pepper and mix until well combined.
2. In a large-sized wok, heat oil over medium heat and cook the turkey mixture for about 8-10 minutes.
3. Add the black beans and tomato and stir to combine.
4. Immediately adjust the heat to low and cook for about 2-3 minutes.
5. Remove the wok of turkey mixture from heat and set aside to cool.
6. Arrange the lettuce leaves onto serving plates.
7. Place the turkey mixture over each lettuce leaf evenly and top with avocado pieces.
8. Garnish with coriander and serve immediately.

Quinoa Lettuce Wraps

Servings|4   Time|15 minutes
Nutritional Content (per serving):
Cal| 119   Fat| 1.7g   Protein| 4.4g   Carbs| 21.7g   Fiber| 3g

Ingredients:

- Cooked quinoa (195 grams)
- Fresh lime juice (5 milliliters)
- Ground black pepper, as required
- Carrot (50 grams, peeled and julienned)
- Green onions (25 grams, chopped)
- Balsamic vinegar (5 milliliters)
- Cucumber (60 grams, peeled and julienned)
- Lettuce leaves (8)

Directions:

1. For filling: in a bowl, add quinoa, Green onions, lime juice, vinegar, black pepper and mix well.
2. Arrange the lettuce leaves onto serving plates.
3. Place quinoa filling over each leaf evenly and top with cucumber and carrot.
4. Serve immediately alongside creamy tofu sauce.

Spinach Soup

Servings|6   Time|1 hour
Nutritional Content (per serving):
Cal| 128   Fat| 7g   Protein| 8.4g   Carbs| 8.7g   Fiber| 1.9g

Ingredients:

- ❖ Olive oil (30 milliliters)
- ❖ Large leeks (2, sliced)
- ❖ Large bunch spinach (1, chopped)
- ❖ Low-fat chicken broth (1920 milliliters)
- ❖ Large onion (1, chopped)
- ❖ Fresh ginger (10 grams, minced)
- ❖ Ground black pepper, as required
- ❖ Fresh lime juice (15 milliliters)

Directions:

1. In a large-sized soup pan, heat oil over low heat and cook the onion and salt for about 20 minutes, stirring occasionally.
2. Stir in the leeks and cook for about 10 minutes.
3. Stir in ginger and spinach and cook for about 5 minutes.
4. Add the broth and stir to combine.
5. Now adjust the heat to medium-high and bring to a boil.
6. Now adjust the heat to medium and cook for about 10 minutes.
7. Remove the soup pan from heat and set aside to cool slightly.
8. In a blender, add the soup mixture and pulse until smooth.
9. Return the soup in the same pan over medium heat and cook for about 5 minutes.
10. Stir in lemon juice and black pepper and serve hot.

Cauliflower Soup

Servings|3   Time|1 hour
Nutritional Content (per serving):
Cal| 93   Fat| 4.7g   Protein| 7g   Carbs| 6.6g   Fiber| 2.7g

Ingredients:

- ❖ Olive oil (15 milliliters)
- ❖ Cauliflower head (1, cut into small florets)
- ❖ Ground black pepper, as required
- ❖ Onion (60 grams, chopped)
- ❖ Fresh ginger (1 (2½-centimeter) piece, chopped)
- ❖ Low-fat chicken broth (720 milliliters)

Directions:

1. In a large-sized soup pan, heat oil over medium heat and sauté the onion for about 1 minute.
2. Add in cauliflower and cook, covered for about 10 minutes, stirring occasionally.
3. Add the remaining ingredients and bring to a rolling full boil.
4. Now adjust the heat to low and simmer, covered for about 30 minutes.
5. Remove from heat and set aside to cool slightly.
6. In a blender, add the soup in 2 batches and pulse until smooth.
7. Return the soup in the same pan over medium-low heat and simmer for about 4-5 minutes or until heated completely.
8. Serve hot.

Avocado Sandwich

Servings|2   Time|10 minutes
Nutritional Content (per serving):
Cal| 225   Fat| 11.3g   Protein| 8.4g   Carbs| 29.3g   Fiber| 7.5g

Ingredients:

- Onion (30 grams, sliced thinly)
- Small avocado (1, peeled, pitted and chopped)
- Dijon mustard (20 grams)
- Tomato (1, sliced)
- Lettuce leaves (4, chopped)
- Whole-wheat bread slices (4, toasted)

Directions:

1. In a large-sized bowl, add the onion, tomato, avocado and lettuce and mix well.
2. Spread Dijon mustard over each bread slice evenly.
3. Divide avocado mixture over 2 slices evenly.
4. Close with remaining 2 slices.
5. With a knife, cut each sandwich in half diagonally and serve.

Tuna Sandwich

Servings|3   Time|10 minutes
Nutritional Content (per serving):
Cal| 243   Fat| 3.5g   Protein| 21.4g   Carbs| 35g   Fiber| 5g

Ingredients:

- Water-packed tuna (1 (150-gram) can, drained)
- Fat-free plain Greek yogurt (70 grams)
- Whole-wheat bread slices (6, toasted)
- Apple (1, peeled, cored and cut into small pieces)
- Mustard (5 grams)
- Honey (10 grams)
- Lettuces leaves (3)

Directions:

1. In a bowl, add the tuna, apple, yogurt, mustard and honey and stir to combine well.
2. Spread the tuna mix over each of 3 bread slices evenly.
3. Top each sandwich with 1 lettuce leaf.
4. Close with the remaining 3 bread slices.
5. With a knife, cut each sandwich in half diagonally and serve.

Chicken Burgers

Servings|4   Time|25 minutes
Nutritional Content (per serving):
Cal| 252   Fat| 13.7g   Protein| 27.4g   Carbs| 5.1g   Fiber| 2.8g

Ingredients:

- Extra-ripe avocado (½, peeled, pitted and cut into chunks
- Garlic clove (1, minced)
- Olive oil cooking spray
- Fresh baby greens (180 grams)
- Low-fat Parmesan cheese (55 grams, grated)
- Ground black pepper, as required

Directions:

1. In a large-sized bowl, add avocado chunks, Parmesan, garlic and black pepper and toss to combine.
2. Add in ground chicken and gently stir to blend.
3. Divide the chicken mixture into 4 equal-sized portions and then shape each into patty.
4. Grease a non-stick grill pan with cooking spray and heat over medium heat.
5. Place the patties into the grill pan and cook for about 4-5 minutes per side.
6. Divide the baby greens onto four serving plates and top each with 1 burger.
7. Serve immediately.

Salmon Burgers

Servings|5   Time|30 minutes
Nutritional Content (per serving):
Cal| 142   Fat| 10.7g   Protein| 9.1g   Carbs| 3.8g   Fiber| 1.3g

Ingredients:

- Canned salmon (155 grams)
- Fresh parsley (5 grams, chopped)
- Paprika (2½ grams)
- Ground black pepper, as required
- Onion (60 grams, minced)
- Garlic clove (1, minced)
- Egg yolks (3)
- Olive oil (30 milliliters)
- Fresh rocket (240 grams)

Directions:

1. Preheat your oven to 180 degrees C.
2. Line a baking sheet with parchment paper.
3. In a large-sized mixing bowl, add all ingredients except for oil and rocket and mix until well combined.
4. Make 10 equal-sized patties from the salmon mixture.
5. Arrange patties onto the prepared baking sheet in a single layer.
6. Bake for approximately 15 minutes.
7. Now, in a large wok, heat oil on high heat.
8. Remove salmon burgers from the oven and transfer into wok.
9. Cook for about 1 minute from both sides.
10. In a bowl, blend together carrot, cabbage, cucumber and Green onions.
11. Divide the rocket onto serving plates and top each with 2 burgers.
12. Serve immediately.

Beef Meatballs

Servings|6 Time|40 minutes
Nutritional Content (per serving):
Cal| 222   Fat| 9.8g   Protein| 25.3g   Carbs| 9g   Fiber| 4.1g

Ingredients:

- Lean ground beef (455 grams)
- Garlic cloves (2, minced)
- Ground cumin (2½ grams)
- Pinch of salt
- Ground black pepper, as required
- Olive oil (30 milliliters)
- Green onions (white part) (25 grams, chopped)
- Red pepper flakes (1¼ grams, crushed)
- Fresh green beans (680 grams, trimmed)

Directions:

1. Preheat your oven to 200 degrees C.
2. Grease a large-sized baking sheet.
3. For meatballs: in a large-sized bowl, add all the ingredients and mix until well combined.
4. Make desired-sized balls from the beef mixture.
5. Arrange the meatballs onto prepared baking sheet in a single layer.
6. Bake for approximately 20-25 minutes or until golden brown.
7. Meanwhile, in a large-sized saucepan of boiling water, add the green beans and cook for about 5-7 minutes.
8. Drain the green beans well and rinse under cold running water.
9. With paper towels, pat dry the beans completely.
10. Transfer the steamed green beans into a large-sized bowl and drizzle with oil.
11. Divide the meatballs onto serving plates and serve alongside the green beans.

Stuffed Courgette

Servings|8   Time|40 minutes
Nutritional Content (per serving):
Cal| 75   Fat| 4.1g   Protein| 3.5g   Carbs| 7.5g   Fiber| 2.2g

Ingredients:

- Medium courgettes (4, halved lengthwise)
- Kalamata olives (85 grams, pitted and minced)
- Garlic clove (1, minced)
- Ground black pepper, as required
- Capsicums (175 grams, seeded and minced)
- Tomatoes (100 grams, finely chopped)
- Dried oregano (5 grams)
- Feta cheese (100 grams, crumbled)

Directions:

1. Preheat your oven to 180 degrees C.
2. Lightly grease a large-sized baking sheet.
3. With a small-sized scooper, scoop out the flesh of each courgette half.
4. In a bowl, add the capsicum, olives, tomatoes, garlic, oregano and black pepper and mix well.
5. Stuff each courgette half with the veggie mixture evenly.
6. Arrange the courgette halves onto prepared baking sheet and bake for approximately 15 minutes.
7. Now, set the oven to broiler on high.
8. Top each Courgette half with feta cheese and broil for about 3 minutes.
9. Serve hot.

Chicken & Broccoli Kabobs

Servings|6   Time|35 minutes
Nutritional Content (per serving):
Cal|231   Fat| 9.3g   Protein| 29g   Carbs| 9.9g   Fiber| 3.7g

Ingredients:

- ❖ Skinless, boneless chicken breasts (680 grams, cubed)
- ❖ Garlic cloves (2, minced)
- ❖ Ground black pepper, as required
- ❖ Olive oil (30 milliliters, divided)
- ❖ Dried marjoram (5 grams)
- ❖ Sugar-free tomato paste (40 grams)
- ❖ Broccoli florets (700 grams)

Directions:

1. In a bowl, add the chicken, 15 milliliters of oil, marjoram, garlic, tomato paste, broccoli and black pepper and mix well.
2. Cover the bowl of chicken and set aside at room temperature for about 10-15 minutes.
3. Thread the chicken and broccoli onto pre-soaked wooden skewers.
4. In a large grill pan, heat remaining oil over medium heat and cook chicken skewers and cook for about 9-10 minutes per side or until desired doneness.
5. Serve hot.

Stuffed Acorn Squash

Servings|4   Time|1 hour 10 minutes
Nutritional Content (per serving):
Cal| 368   Fat| 13.9g   Protein| 33.4g   Carbs| 31g   Fiber| 6g

Ingredients:

- Acorn squash (2, halved and seeded)
- Onion (60 grams, chopped)
- Fresh mushrooms (100 grams, sliced)
- Sugar-free tomato sauce (225 grams)
- Low-fat cheddar cheese (115 grams, shredded)
- Lean ground turkey (455 grams)
- Celery stalk (200 grams, chopped)
- Dried oregano (5 grams)
- Dried basil 5 grams
- Ground black pepper, as required

Directions:

1. Preheat your oven to 180 degrees C.
2. In the bottom of a microwave-safe glass baking dish, arrange the squash halves, cut side down.
3. Microwave on high power for about 19-20 minutes or until almost tender.
4. Heat a large non-stick wok over medium heat and cook the ground turkey for about 4-5 minutes or until browned. Drain the grease.
5. In the wok, add the onion and celery and cook for about 3-4 minutes.
6. Stir in mushrooms and cook for about 2-3 minutes more.
7. Stir in the tomato sauce, dried herbs and black pepper and remove from heat.
8. Spoon the turkey mixture into each squash half.
9. Cover the baking dish and transfer into the oven.
10. Bake for approximately 15 minutes.
11. Uncover the baking dish and sprinkle each squash half with cheddar cheese.
12. Bake, uncovered for approximately 3-5 minutes or until the cheese becomes bubbly.
13. Serve hot.

Lemony Shrimp

Servings|3   Time|23 minutes
Nutritional Content (per serving):
Cal| 270   Fat| 11.3g   Protein| 34.9g   Carbs| 4.3g   Fiber| 0.4g

Ingredients:

- Olive oil (30 milliliters)
- Garlic cloves (3, minced)
- Lemon (1, sliced thinly)
- Pinch of salt
- Water (30 milliliters)
- Fresh parsley (5 grams, chopped)

- Medium shrimp (455 grams, peeled and deveined)
- Red pepper flakes (1½ grams, crushed)
- Fresh lemon juice (15 milliliters)

Directions:

1. In a large-sized wok, heat oil over medium heat and cook the shrimp, garlic, lemon slices, red pepper flakes and salt for about 3 minutes per side, stirring occasionally.
2. Stir in the water, lemon juice and parsley and immediately remove from heat.
3. Serve hot.

Dinner Recipes

Steak & Peach Salad

Servings|4   Time|27 minutes
Nutritional Content (per serving):
Cal| 361   Fat| 18.1g   Protein| 34.8g   Carbs| 14.8g   Fiber| 2.7g

Ingredients:

- ❖ Fresh lemon juice (15 milliliters, pinch of salt
- ❖ Ground black pepper, as required
- ❖ Olive oil cooking spray
- ❖ Fresh baby rocket (240 grams)
- ❖ Peaches (3, pitted and sliced)
- ❖ Extra-virgin olive oil (15 milliliters, divided)
- ❖ Flank steak (455 grams, trimmed)
- ❖ Maple syrup (10 grams)
- ❖ Feta cheese (30 grams, crumbled)

Directions:

1. In a large-sized bowl, blend together 5 milliliters of lemon juice, 5 milliliters of oil, salt and black pepper.
2. Add the steak and coat with mixture generously.
3. Grease a non-stick wok with cooking spray and heat over medium-high heat.
4. In the wok, add the steak and cook for about 5-6 minutes per side.
5. Place the steak onto a platter for about 9-10 minutes before slicing.
6. Cut the steak into desired-sized slices diagonally across the grain.
7. In a large-sized bowl, add the remaining lemon juice, oil, maple syrup, salt and black pepper and beat until well combined.
8. Add the rocket and toss to coat well.
9. Divide the rocket onto 4 serving plates.
10. Top with steak slices, peach slices and cheese evenly and serve.

Quinoa & Mango Salad

Servings|4   Time|15 minutes
Nutritional Content (per serving):
Cal| 380   Fat| 18g   Protein| 9.9g   Carbs| 51.6g   Fiber| 8.4g

Ingredients:

- Cooked quinoa (370 grams)
- Avocado (1, peeled, pitted and chopped)
- Fresh baby rocket (60 grams)
- Garlic cloves (2, minced)
- Olive oil (20 milliliters)
- Salt, as required
- Mango (250 grams, peeled, pitted, and chopped)
- Radishes (115 grams, sliced)
- Fresh mint (10 grams, chopped)
- Fresh lemon juice (30 milliliters)

Directions:

1. In a large-sized salad bowl, add all ingredients and gently stir to combine.
2. Refrigerate for about 1-2 hours before serving.

Chicken Taco Bowl

Servings|4   Time|30 minutes
Nutritional Content (per serving):
Cal| 352   Fat| 17.8g   Protein| 34.6g   Carbs| 15.9g   Fiber| 6.9g

Ingredients:

- Boneless, skinless chicken breasts (4 (115-gram))
- Olive oil (30 milliliters)
- Cooked black beans (170 grams)
- Large avocado (1, peeled, pitted and sliced)
- Green onions (2, chopped)
- Fresh coriander (5 grams, chopped)
- Pinch of salt
- Ground black pepper, as required
- Low-fat chicken broth (180 milliliters)
- Large tomato (1, chopped)
- Jalapeño pepper (½, chopped)
- Low-fat cheddar cheese (30 grams, shredded)

Directions:

1. Rub each chicken breast with salt and black pepper evenly.
2. In a large-sized wok, heat oil over medium heat and cook the chicken breasts for about 5 minutes.
3. Flip the chicken breast and top with the broth.
4. Cook, covered for about 7-10 minutes or until cooked through.
5. With a slotted spoon, transfer the chicken breast into a bowl and with 2 forks, shred the meat.
6. Add any remaining liquid from the pan into the shredded chicken and stir to combine.
7. Divide the shredded chicken into serving bowls and serve with the topping of remaining ingredients.

Lemony Chicken Breasts

Servings|4   Time|24 minutes
Nutritional Content (per serving):
Cal| 292   Fat| 11.7g   Protein| 43.5g   Carbs| 0.5g   Fiber| 0.1g

Ingredients:

- Balsamic vinegar (60 milliliters)
- Boneless, skinless chicken breasts (4 (150-gram), pounded slightly)
- Olive oil (30 milliliters)
- Fresh lime juice (15 milliliters)
- Lemon-pepper seasoning (1½ grams)

Directions:

1. In a glass baking dish, add vinegar, oil, lemon juice and seasoning and mix until well blended.
2. Add the chicken breasts and coat with the mixture generously.
3. Refrigerate to marinate for about 25-30 minutes.
4. Preheat the grill to medium heat. Grease the grill grate.
5. Remove the chicken breasts from bowl and discard the remaining marinade.
6. Place the chicken breasts onto the grill and cover with the lid.
7. Cook for about 5-7 minutes per side.
8. Serve hot.

Parmesan Chicken Bake

Servings|4   Time|55 minutes
Nutritional Content (per serving):
Cal| 300   Fat| 11.3g   Protein| 43.5g   Carbs| 3.8g   Fiber| 0.1g

Ingredients:

- ❖ Fat-free plain Greek yogurt (280 grams)
- ❖ Garlic powder (2½ grams)
- ❖ Ground black pepper, as required
- ❖ Low-fat Parmesan cheese (55 grams, grated)
- ❖ Boneless, skinless chicken breasts (4 (115-gram))

Directions:

1. Preheat your oven to 190 degrees C.
2. Line baking sheet with a greased piece of foil.
3. In a bowl, add the yogurt, cheese, garlic powder and black pepper and mix until well blended.
4. Add the chicken breasts and coat with yogurt mixture evenly.
5. Arrange the chicken breasts onto the prepared baking sheet in a single layer.
6. Bake for approximately 45 minutes.
7. Serve hot.

Ground Turkey Chili

Servings|8   Time|2½ hours
Nutritional Content (per serving):
Cal| 254   Fat| 12.9g   Protein| 25.9g   Carbs| 11.2g   Fiber| 3g

Ingredients:

- Olive oil (30 milliliters)
- Large capsicum (1, seeded and chopped)
- Dried thyme (5 grams)
- Ground cumin (10 grams)
- Tomatoes (400 grams, finely chopped)
- Sugar-free tomato paste (1 (150-gram) can)
- Green onions (4, chopped)
- Large onion (1, chopped)
- Garlic cloves (4, minced)
- Jalapeño pepper (1, chopped)
- Red chili powder (10 grams)
- Lean ground turkey (910 grams)
- Low-fat chicken broth (480 milliliters)
- Water (240 milliliters)

Directions:

1. In a large-sized soup pan, heat oil over medium heat and sauté the onion and capsicum for about 5-7 minutes.
2. Add the garlic, jalapeño pepper, dried herbs, spices and black pepper and sauté for about 1 minute.
3. Add the turkey and cook for about 4-5 minutes.
4. Stir in the tomatoes, tomato paste and cacao powder and cook for about 2 minutes.
5. Add in broth and water and bring to a rolling full boil.
6. Now adjust the heat to low and simmer, covered for about 2 hours.
7. Serve hot with the garnishing of Green onions.

Beef with Cauliflower

Servings|4   Time|27 minutes
Nutritional Content (per serving):
Cal| 271   Fat| 10.9g   Protein| 36.8g   Carbs| 5.7g   Fiber| 2.3g

Ingredients:

- ❖ Extra-virgin olive oil (15 milliliters)
- ❖ Beef sirloin steak (455 grams, cut into bite-sized pieces)
- ❖ Pinch of salt
- ❖ ground black pepper, as required
- ❖ Garlic cloves (2, minced)
- ❖ Cauliflower florets (350 grams)
- ❖ Low-fat chicken broth (60 milliliters)
- ❖ Fresh coriander (5 grams, chopped)

Directions:

1. In a large-sized wok, heat olive oil over medium heat and sauté the garlic for about 1 minute.
2. Add the beef pieces and stir to combine.
3. Increase the heat to medium-high and cook for about 6-8 minutes or until browned from all sides.
4. Meanwhile, in a pan of boiling water, add the cauliflower and cook for about 5-6 minutes.
5. Remove the pan from heat and drain the cauliflower completely.
6. Add the cauliflower and broth in sauté pan with beef and cook for about 2-3 minutes.
7. Stir in the black pepper and remove from heat.
8. Serve hot with the garnishing of coriander.

Beef & Pumpkin Stew

Servings|4   Time|2 hours 25 minutes
Nutritional Content (per serving):
Cal| 361   Fat| 13.9g   Protein| 27.8g   Carbs| 20.3g   Fiber| 6.6g

Ingredients:

- Beef stew meat (455 grams, trimmed and cubed)
- Extra-virgin olive oil (30 milliliters, divided)
- Celery stalks (2, chopped)
- Pumpkin (500 grams, peeled and cubed)
- Fresh coriander (10 grams, chopped)
- Pinch of salt
- Ground black pepper, as required
- Carrot (1, peeled and finely chopped)
- Onion (1, chopped)
- Tomatoes (600 grams, finely chopped)
- Water (960 milliliters)

Directions:

1. Sprinkle the beef cubes with salt and black pepper evenly.
2. In a large saucepan, heat 15 milliliters of oil over medium heat and sear beef for about 4-5 minutes.
3. Transfer the beef into a large-sized bowl and set aside.
4. In the same pan, heat the remaining oil over medium heat and sauté carrot, celery and onion for about 5 minutes.
5. Add pumpkin and tomatoes and sauté for about 5 minutes.
6. Add water and beef and bring to a boil over high heat.
7. Now adjust the heat to low and simmer, covered for about 1 hour.
8. Uncover and simmer for about 50 minutes.
9. Serve hot with the garnishing of coriander.

Pork Chops in Sauce

Servings|4   Time|25 minutes
Nutritional Content (per serving):
Cal| 343   Fat| 21g   Protein| 31g   Carbs| 3.2g   Fiber| 0.2g

Ingredients:

- Garlic cloves (2, chopped)
- Fresh coriander (5 grams)
- Fresh lime juice (30 milliliters)
- Unsweetened coconut milk (380 milliliters)
- Coconut oil (15 grams)
- Jalapeño pepper (1, chopped)
- Ground turmeric (1½ grams, divided)
- Pork chops (4)
- Pinch of salt
- Shallot (1, finely chopped)

Directions:

1. In a blender, add garlic, jalapeño pepper, coriander, turmeric, lime juice and coconut milk and pulse until smooth.
2. Sprinkle the pork with salt and remaining turmeric evenly.
3. In a sauté pan, melt coconut oil over medium-high heat and sauté shallots for about 1 minute.
4. Add in pork chops and cook for about 2 minutes per side.
5. Transfer the chops into a bowl.
6. Add in coconut milk mixture and bring to a boil.
7. Now adjust the heat to medium and simmer for about 5 minutes, stirring occasionally.
8. Stir in pork chops and cook for about 3-5 minutes.
9. Serve hot.

Cod with Olives & Tomatoes

Servings|4   Time|30 minutes
Nutritional Content (per serving):
Cal| 215   Fat| 10.9g   Protein| 22.8g   Carbs| 8.4g   Fiber| 2.5g

Ingredients:

- Extra-virgin olive oil (30 milliliters)
- Low-fat chicken broth (180 milliliters)
- Black olives (85 grams, pitted and sliced)
- Cod fillets (455 grams)
- Onion (1, sliced thinly)
- Garlic cloves (2, minced)
- Fresh parsley (5 grams, chopped)
- Tomatoes (400 grams, finely chopped)

Directions:

1. In a large-sized wok, heat oil over medium heat and sauté the onion and garlic for about 4-5 minutes.
2. Add the remaining ingredients except for cod fillets and cook for about 5 minutes.
3. Stir in the cod fillets and cook for about 5 minutes or until desired doneness.
4. Serve hot.

Salmon Soup

Servings|8   Time|1 hour 25 minutes
Nutritional Content (per serving):
Cal| 286   Fat| 13.4g   Protein| 20.4g   Carbs| 22.2g   Fiber| 4.1g

Ingredients:

- ❖ Onions (240 grams, chopped)
- ❖ Garlic cloves (2, chopped)
- ❖ Fresh ginger root (10 grams, finely chopped)
- ❖ Quinoa (190 grams, rinsed)
- ❖ Salmon fillets (400 grams)
- ❖ Fresh baby spinach (180 grams)
- ❖ Fresh coriander (20 grams, chopped)
- ❖ Celery stalk (200 grams, chopped)
- ❖ Fresh mushrooms (100 grams, sliced)
- ❖ Low-fat chicken broth (1920 milliliters)
- ❖ Unsweetened coconut milk (240 milliliters)
- ❖ Salt, as required

Directions:

1. In a large-sized soup pan, add onions, celery stalk, garlic, ginger root, mushrooms, quinoa and broth and bring to a boil.
2. Now adjust the heat to low and simmer, covered for about 45 minutes.
3. Arrange the halibut fillets over the soup mixture.
4. Simmer, covered for about 15 minutes.
5. Stir in remaining ingredients and simmer for about 5 minutes.
6. Serve hot.

Shrimp & Tomato Bake

Servings|6   Time|40 minutes
Nutritional Content (per serving):
Cal| 249   Fat| 11.3g   Protein| 30.1g   Carbs| 6.4g   Fiber| 1.4g

Ingredients:

- Extra-virgin olive oil (30 milliliters)
- Dried oregano (5 grams, crushed)
- Fresh parsley (15 grams, chopped)
- Fresh lemon juice (15 milliliters)
- Feta cheese (115 grams, crumbled)
- Garlic cloves (2, minced)
- Shrimp (680 grams, peeled and deveined)
- Red pepper flakes (2½ grams, crushed)
- Low-fat chicken broth (180 milliliters)
- Tomatoes (400 grams, chopped

Directions:

1. Preheat your oven to 180 degrees C.
2. In a large-sized wok, heat oil over medium-high heat and sauté the garlic for about 1 minute.
3. Add the shrimp, oregano and red pepper flakes and cook for about 4-5 minutes.
4. Stir in the parsley and immediately remove from heat.
5. Transfer the shrimp mixture into a casserole dish and spread in an even layer.
6. In the same wok, add the broth and lemon juice over medium heat and simmer for about 3-5 minutes or until reduced to half.
7. Stir in the tomatoes and cook for about 2-3 minutes.
8. Remove from heat and place the tomato mixture over shrimp mixture evenly.
9. Top with feta cheese evenly.
10. Bake for approximately 16-20 minutes or until top becomes golden brown.
11. Serve hot.

Beans & Sweet Potato Chili

Servings|4   Time|2½ hours
Nutritional Content (per serving):
Cal| 312   Fat| 10.3g   Protein| 12.8g   Carbs| 48.6g   Fiber| 12g

Ingredients:

- Olive oil (30 milliliters)
- Small capsicums (2, seeded and chopped)
- Red chili powder (10-15 grams)
- Tomatoes (600 grams, finely chopped)
- Canned corn kernels (165 grams)
- Ground black pepper, as required
- Onion (, chopped)
- Garlic cloves (4, minced)
- Ground cumin (5 grams)
- Medium sweet potato (1, peeled and chopped)
- Canned red kidney beans (350 grams
- Low-fat vegetable broth (480 milliliters)
- Pinch of salt

Directions:

1. In a large-sized soup pan, heat oil over medium-high heat and sauté onion and capsicums for about 3-4 minutes.
2. Add garlic and spices and sauté for 1 minute.
3. Add sweet potato and cook for about 4-5 minutes.
4. Add remaining all ingredients and bring to a boil.
5. Now adjust the heat to medium-low and simmer, covered for about 1-2 hours.
6. Season with salt and black pepper and serve hot.

Chickpeas & Pumpkin Curry

Servings|5   Time|50 minutes
Nutritional Content (per serving):
Cal| 204   Fat| 5g   Protein| 8.6g   Carbs| 34.7g   Fiber| 5.9g

Ingredients:

- Olive oil (15 milliliters)
- Garlic cloves (2, minced)
- Ground cumin (5 grams)
- Ground coriander (2½ grams)
- Tomatoes (400 grams, finely chopped)
- Low-fat vegetable broth (480 milliliters)
- Pinch of salt
- Ground black pepper, as required
- Onion (1, chopped)
- Green chili (1, seeded and finely chopped)
- Red chili powder (5 grams)
- Pumpkin (910 grams, peeled and cubed)
- Canned chickpeas (350 grams, rinsed and drained)
- Fresh coriander leaves (10 grams, chopped)
- Fresh lime juice (30 milliliters)

Directions:

1. In a large-sized saucepan, heat oil over medium-high heat and sauté onion for about 5-7 minutes.
2. Add garlic, green chili and spices and sauté for about 1 minute.
3. Add tomatoes and cook for 2-3 minutes, crushing with the back of the spoon.
4. Add pumpkin and cook for about 3-4 minutes, stirring occasionally.
5. Add broth and bring to a boil.
6. Now adjust the heat to low and simmer for about 10 minutes.
7. Stir in chickpeas and simmer for about 10 minutes.
8. Stir in salt, black pepper and lemon juice and serve hot with the garnishing of coriander.

Lentils & Quinoa Stew

Servings|6   Time|48 minutes
Nutritional Content (per serving):
Cal| 291   Fat| 5.5g   Protein| 17.7g   Carbs| 44g   Fiber| 14.3g

Ingredients:

- Olive oil (15 milliliters)
- Onion (1, chopped)
- Tomatoes (800 grams, chopped)
- Quinoa (95 grams, rinsed)
- Red chili powder (5 grams)
- Low-fat vegetable broth (1200 milliliters)
- Carrots (3, peeled and chopped)
- Celery stalks (3, chopped)
- Garlic cloves (4, minced)
- Red lentils (210 grams, rinsed and drained)
- Ground cumin (5 grams)
- Fresh spinach (60 grams, chopped)

Directions:

1. In a large-sized soup pan, heat oil over medium heat and cook the celery, onion and carrot for about 8 minutes, stirring frequently.
2. Add the garlic and sauté for about 50-60 seconds.
3. Add the remaining ingredients except for spinach and bring to a boil.
4. Now adjust the heat to low and simmer, covered for about 20 minutes.
5. Stir in spinach and simmer for about 3-4 minutes.
6. Serve hot.

Snack Recipes

Cheese & Strawberry Bowl

Servings|2 Time|5 minutes
Nutritional Content (per serving):
Cal| 37   Fat| 0.7g   Protein| 4.3g   Carbs| 3.6g   Fiber| 0.7g

Ingredients:

- 1 Low-fat cottage cheese (60 grams)
- Fresh strawberries (65 grams, hulled and sliced)

Directions:

1. In a bowl, add all ingredients and stir to combine.
2. Serve immediately.

Roasted Almonds

Servings|4 Time|10 minutes
Nutritional Content (per serving):
Cal| 200   Fat| 16.3g   Protein| 6.4g   Carbs| 6.6g   Fiber| 4g

Ingredients:

- Whole almonds (140 grams)
- Ground black pepper, as required
- Ground cinnamon (1¼ grams)
- Extra-virgin olive oil (10 milliliters)

Directions:

1. Preheat your oven to 180 degrees C.
2. Line a baking dish with parchment paper.
3. In a bowl, add all ingredients and toss to coat well.
4. Transfer the almond mixture into the prepared baking dish and spread in a single layer.
5. Roast for about 10 minutes, flipping twice.
6. Remove the baking dish of walnuts from oven and set aside to cool completely before serving.

Roasted Cashews

Servings|8   Time|20 minutes
Nutritional Content (per serving):
Cal| 191   Fat| 14.4g   Protein| 5.9g   Carbs| 9.6g   Fiber| 1.2g

Ingredients:

- ❖ Cashews (260 grams)
- ❖ Fresh lime juice (15 milliliters)
- ❖ Ground cumin (2½ grams)
- ❖ Cayenne pepper (1¼ grams)

Directions:

1. Preheat your oven to 200 degrees C.
2. Line a roasting pan with a heavy-duty sheet of foil.
3. In a large-sized bowl, add the cashews and spices and toss to coat well.
4. Transfer the cashews into the prepared roasting pan.
5. Roast for about 8-10 minutes.
6. Drizzle with lime juice and serve.

Carrot Sticks

Servings|8   Time|35 minutes
Nutritional Content (per serving):
Cal| 22   Fat| 0g   Protein| 0.4g   Carbs| 5.3g   Fiber| 1.3g

Ingredients:

- ❖ Large carrots (6, peeled and cut into 2-inch long sticks)
- ❖ Olive oil cooking spray

Directions:

1. Preheat your oven to 200 degrees C.
2. Lightly grease 2 large-sized baking sheets.
3. Arrange carrot sticks onto prepared baking sheets and spray with cooking spray.
4. Roast for approximately 20 minutes.
5. Serve warm.

Cauliflower Poppers

Servings|4   Time|40 minutes
Nutritional Content (per serving):
Cal| 43   Fat| 2.5g   Protein| 1.8g   Carbs| 4.8g   Fiber| 2.3g

Ingredients:

- Cauliflower florets (350 grams)
- Red chili powder (1¼ grams)
- Pinch of salt
- Olive oil (15 milliliters)
- Ground black pepper, as required

Directions:

1. Preheat your oven to 230 degrees C.
2. Grease a roasting pan.
3. In a bowl, add all ingredients and toss to coat well.
4. Transfer the cauliflower mixture into the prepared roasting pan and spread in an even layer.
5. Roast for approximately 25-30 minutes.
6. Serve warm.

Sweet Potato Croquettes

Servings|4   Time|45 minutes
Nutritional Content (per serving):
Cal| 251   Fat| 15.5g   Protein| 9.8g   Carbs| 21.3g   Fiber| 5.8g

Ingredients:

- Cooked sweet potato (300 grams, peeled and chopped roughly)
- Almond meal (100 grams)
- Almond butter (30 grams)
- Pinch of salt
- Eggs (2)

Directions:

1. Preheat your oven to 200 degrees C.
2. Line a large-sized baking sheet with lightly greased parchment paper.
3. In a bowl, add the sweet potato and with a fork mash it.
4. Add the almond butter and salt and mix well.
5. In a shallow dish, crack the eggs and beat well.
6. In another shallow dish, place the almond meal.
7. With a tablespoon of the sweet potato mixture, make balls and flatten each slightly.
8. Dip the croquettes in beaten eggs and then roll in almond meal completely.
9. Arrange the croquettes onto the prepared baking sheet in a single layer.
10. Bake for approximately 25-30 minutes or until done completely.
11. Serve warm.

Almond Scones

Servings|6 Time|35 minutes
Nutritional Content (per serving):
Cal| 239 Fat| 19.6g   Protein| 3.8g   Carbs| 13.1g   Fiber| 2.8g

Ingredients:

- Almonds (70 grams)
- Arrowroot flour (30 grams)
- Ground turmeric (5 grams)
- Ground black pepper, as required
- Organic vanilla extract (5 milliliters)

- Almonds flour (140 grams)
- Coconut flour (5 grams)
- Pinch of salt
- Egg (1)
- Olive oil (60 milliliters)
- Honey (55 grams)

Directions:

1. Preheat your oven to 180 degrees C.
2. Lightly grease a baking sheet.
3. In a food processor, add the almonds and pulse until chopped roughly
4. Transfer the chopped almonds into a large-sized bowl.
5. Add the flours, turmeric, salt and black pepper and mix well.
6. In another bowl, add remaining ingredients and beat until well combined.
7. Add the flour mixture into egg mixture and mix until well combined.
8. Arrange a plastic wrap over a cutting board.
9. Place the dough over a cutting board.
10. With your hands, pat the dough into about 2½-centimeter thick circle.
11. Carefully cut the circle in 6 wedges.
12. Arrange the scones onto the prepared baking sheet in a single layer.
13. Bake for approximately 15-20 minutes.
14. Serve warm.

Fish Sticks

Servings|6   Time|35 minutes
Nutritional Content (per serving):
Cal| 220   Fat| 12.1g   Protein| 24.3g   Carbs| 3.3g   Fiber| 1.2g

Ingredients:

- Tilapia fillets (455 grams, cut into strips)
- Low-fat Parmesan cheese (125 grams, shredded)
- Almond flour (100 grams)
- Ground black pepper, as required
- Large eggs (2, beaten)

Directions:

1. Preheat your oven to 230 degrees C. Line a baking sheet with parchment paper.
2. In a shallow bowl, add the flour and black pepper and mix until well combined.
3. In a second shallow bowl, add a splash of water and eggs and beat well.
4. In a third shallow bowl, place the cheese.
5. Coat the tilapia strips with the flour mixture, then dip into the beaten eggs and finally coat with the cheese.
6. Arrange the coated tilapia strips onto prepared baking sheet in a single layer.
7. Bake for approximately 18-20 minutes or until done completely.
8. Remove from heat and serve warm.

Deviled Eggs

Servings|4   Time|35 minutes
Nutritional Content (per serving):
Cal| 174   Fat| 14.8g   Protein| 7.2g   Carbs| 4.7g   Fiber| 3.4g

Ingredients:

- Large eggs (4)
- Fresh lime juice (10 milliliters)
- Pinch of salt
- Medium avocado (1, peeled, pitted and chopped)
- Pinch of cayenne pepper

Directions:

1. In a pan of water, add the eggs and cook for about 15-20 minutes.
2. Remove from heat and drain the eggs.
3. Set aside to cool completely.
4. Peel each boiled egg and then cut in half vertically.
5. Carefully scoop out the yolks from each egg half.
6. In a bowl, add half of the egg yolks, avocado, lime juice and salt and with a fork, mash until well combined.
7. Spoon the avocado mixture in each egg half evenly.
8. Serve with the sprinkling of cayenne pepper.

Blueberry Bites

Servings|10   Time|15 minutes
Nutritional Content (per serving):
Cal| 36   Fat| 0.8g   Protein| 3.3g   Carbs| 4g   Fiber| 2.2g

Ingredients:

- Unsweetened protein powder (30 grams)
- Ground cinnamon (1¼ grams)
- Unsweetened almond milk (120-240 milliliters)
- Coconut flour (45 grams, sifted)
- Powdered Erythritol (10-20 grams)
- Dried blueberries (40-45 grams)

Directions:

1. Line a large-sized cookie sheet with parchment paper. Set aside.
2. In a large-sized bowl, add all the ingredients except almond milk and mix well.
3. Gradually add desired amount of almond milk and mix until dough forms.
4. Immediately, make desired-sized balls from mixture.
5. Arrange the blueberry balls onto the prepared baking sheet in a single layer.
6. Refrigerate to set for about 30 minutes before serving.

Quinoa Crackers

Servings|6   Time|35 minutes
Nutritional Content (per serving):
Cal| 40   Fat| 2.9g   Protein| 1.5g   Carbs| 3.1g   Fiber| 1.2g

Ingredients:

- ❖ Water (45 milliliters)
- ❖ Sunflower seeds (25 grams)
- ❖ Ground turmeric (5 grams)
- ❖ Chia seeds (10 grams)
- ❖ Quinoa flour (10 grams)
- ❖ Pinch of sea salt

Directions:

1. Preheat your oven to 175 degrees C.
2. Line a baking sheet with parchment paper.
3. In a bowl, add the water and chia seeds and soak for about 15 minutes.
4. After 15 minutes, add remaining ingredients and mix well.
5. Place the seeds mixture onto the prepared baking sheet and with the back of a spoon, smooth the top surface.
6. With a knife, cut the dough into small-sized crackers.
7. Bake for approximately 20 minutes.
8. Remove the baking sheet of crackers from oven and set aside to cool completely before serving.

Brinjal Caviar

Servings|4   Time|35 minutes
Nutritional Content (per serving):
Cal| 110   Fat| 4.1g   Protein| 3.2g   Carbs| 18.4g   Fiber| 10.4g

Ingredients:

- Brinjals (1135 grams, halved lengthwise)
- Fresh basil leaves (5 grams)
- Fresh lemon juice (15 milliliters)
- Garlic cloves (2, chopped)
- Green onions (50 grams, chopped)
- Low-fat vegetable broth (30 milliliters)
- Olive oil (15 milliliters)

Directions:

1. Preheat your oven to 200 degrees C.
2. Grease a baking sheet.
3. Place brinjal halves onto the prepared baking sheet, cut-side facing down.
4. Roast for about 20 minutes.
5. Remove the baking sheet of brinjal from the oven and let them cool slightly.
6. With a small-sized spoon, scoop out the pulp from skin.
7. In a food processor, add brinjal pulp and remaining ingredients except for oil and pulse until smooth.
8. Transfer the caviar into a bowl.
9. Add the olive oil and stir to combine.
10. Serve at room temperature.

Black Beans Hummus

Servings|10   Time|15 minutes
Nutritional Content (per serving):
Cal| 197   Fat| 4.2g   Protein| 11.7g   Carbs| 30.1g   Fiber| 11g

Ingredients:

- Canned black beans (1140 grams, rinsed and drained)
- Tahini (55 grams)
- Hot sauce (5 milliliters)
- Salsa (60 grams)
- Garlic cloves (2, chopped)
- Boiled cauliflower (200 grams)
- Olive oil (5 milliliters)

Directions:

1. Add all ingredients in a high-power blender and pulse until smooth.
2. Transfer into a bowl and serve.

Berries Gazpacho

Servings|6   Time|15 minutes
Nutritional Content (per serving):
Cal| 86   Fat| 2.9g   Protein| 1.7g   Carbs| 15.6g   Fiber| 4.9g

Ingredients:

- Fresh raspberries (250 grams)
- Unsweetened almond milk (960 milliliters)
- Fresh blueberries (380 grams)
- Organic vanilla extract (2½ milliliters)

Directions:

1. In a clean food processor, add the ingredients and pulse until smooth.
2. Serve immediately.

Air Fry Recipes

Pumpkin & Yogurt Bread

Servings|4   Time|25 minutes
Nutritional Content (per serving):
Cal| 175   Fat| 3.1g   Protein| 7g   Carbs| 27.8g   Fiber| 1.8g

Ingredients:

- Large eggs (2)
- Banana flour (50 grams)
- Honey (70 grams)
- Organic vanilla extract (15 milliliters)
- Gluten-free oats (35-40 grams)
- Sugar-free pumpkin puree (115 grams)
- Fat-free plain Greek yogurt (70 grams)
- Pinch of ground nutmeg

Directions:

1. Grease and flour a loaf pan. Set aside.
2. In a bowl, add all ingredients except for oats and with a hand mixer, mix until smooth.
3. Add the oats and mix well.
4. Place the bread mixture into prepared loaf pan evenly.
5. Set the temperature of Air Fryer to 185 degrees C to preheat for 5 minutes.
6. After preheating, arrange the loaf pan into an Air Fryer Basket.
7. Slide the basket into Air Fryer and set the time for 15 minutes.
8. After cooking time is finished, remove the loaf pan from Air Fryer and place onto a wire rack for about 10 minutes.
9. Remove the bread from pan and place onto the wire rack to cool completely before slicing.
10. Cut the bread into desired-sized slices and serve.

Mushroom & Tomato Frittata

Servings|2   Time|15 minutes
Nutritional Content (per serving):
Cal| 249   Fat| 19.4g   Protein| 16.3g   Carbs| 4g   Fiber| 1.1g

Ingredients:

- ❖ Olive oil (15 milliliters)
- ❖ Fresh mushrooms (8, sliced)
- ❖ Low-fat Parmesan cheese (55 grams, grated)
- ❖ Cherry tomatoes (6, halved)
- ❖ Eggs (3)
- ❖ Fresh parsley (5 grams, chopped)

Directions:

1. Set the temperature of Air Fryer to 195 degrees C to preheat for 5 minutes.
2. In a baking dish, blend together the tomatoes, mushrooms, salt, and black pepper.
3. After preheating, arrange the baking dish into an Air Fryer Basket.
4. Slide the basket into Air Fryer and set the time for 14 minutes.
5. Meanwhile, in a small-sized bowl, add the eggs and beat well.
6. Add in the parsley and cheese and mix well.
7. After 6 minutes of cooking, top the mushroom mixture with egg mixture.
8. After cooking time is finished, remove the baking dish from Air Fryer and serve hot.

Glazed Chicken Drumsticks

Servings|4   Time|32 minutes
Nutritional Content (per serving):
Cal| 280   Fat| 17.3g   Protein| 23.2g   Carbs| 6.8g   Fiber| 1.7g

Ingredients:

- Dijon mustard (80 grams)
- Fresh rosemary (5 grams, minced)
- 4 (150-grams) boneless chicken drumsticks
- Honey (20 grams)
- Fresh thyme (5 grams, minced)
- Pinch of salt
- Ground black pepper, as required

Directions:

1. In a large-sized bowl, blend together the mustard, honey, oil, herbs, salt and black pepper.
2. Add the drumsticks and coat with the mixture generously.
3. Cover and refrigerate to marinate overnight.
4. Set the temperature of Air Fryer to 160 degrees C to preheat for 5 minutes.
5. After preheating, arrange the chicken drumsticks into the greased Air Fryer Basket in a single layer.
6. Slide the basket into Air Fryer and set the time for 12 minutes.
7. After 12 minutes of cooking, set the temperature to 180 degrees C for 8-10 minutes.
8. After cooking time is finished, remove the drumsticks from Air Fryer and serve hot.

Spiced Chicken Breasts

Servings|4   Time|33 minutes
Nutritional Content (per serving):
Cal| 225   Fat| 9.2g   Protein| 35g   Carbs| 0.6g   Fiber| 0.2g

Ingredients:

- Olive oil (30 milliliters)
- Pinch of salt
- Skinless, boneless chicken breasts (4 (150-grams))
- Smoked paprika (1¼ grams
- Ground black pepper, as required

Directions:

1. In a bowl, blend together oil, paprika, salt and black pepper.
2. Coat the chicken breasts with the oil mixture evenly.
3. Set the temperature of Air Fryer to 180 degrees C to preheat for 5 minutes.
4. After preheating, arrange chicken breasts into the greased Air Fryer Basket in a single layer.
5. Slide the basket into Air Fryer and set the time for 20-23 minutes.
6. After 15 minutes of cooking, flip chicken breasts once.
7. After cooking time is finished, remove chicken breasts from Air Fryer and serve hot.

Herbed Turkey Breast

Servings|6   Time|45 minutes
Nutritional Content (per serving):
Cal| 351   Fat| 16.1g   Protein| 40.7g   Carbs| 2.2g   Fiber| 0.8g

Ingredients:

- Dried thyme (5 grams)
- Paprika (1½ grams)
- Ground black pepper, as required
- Olive oil (15 milliliters)

- Dried rosemary (5 grams)
- Pinch of salt
- Bone-in, skin-on turkey breast (1135 gram)

Directions:

1. In a bowl, blend together the herbs, paprika, salt and black pepper.
2. Coat the turkey breast with oil and then rub with herb mixture.
3. Set the temperature of Air Fryer to 185 degrees C to preheat for 5 minutes.
4. After preheating, arrange the turkey breast into the greased Air Fryer Basket, skin-side down.
5. Slide the basket into Air Fryer and set the time for 35 minutes.
6. While cooking, flip the turkey breast once halfway through.
7. After cooking time is finished, remove the turkey breast from Air Fryer and place onto a cutting board for about 9-10 minutes before slicing.
8. Cut the turkey breast into desired-sized slices and serve.

Simple Filet Mignon

Servings|2   Time|24 minutes
Nutritional Content (per serving):
Cal| 300   Fat| 17.7g   Protein| 33.2g   Carbs| 0g   Fiber| 0g

Ingredients:

- Filet mignon steaks (2 (150-grams))
- Pinch of salt
- Olive oil (15 milliliters)
- Ground black pepper, as required

Directions:

1. Coat each steak with oil and then season with salt and black pepper.
2. Set the temperature of Air Fryer to 195 degrees C to preheat for 5 minutes.
3. After preheating, arrange the steaks into the greased Air Fryer Basket.
4. Slide the basket into Air Fryer and set the time for 14 minutes.
5. While cooking, flip the filets once halfway through.
6. After cooking time is finished, remove the steaks from Air Fryer and serve hot.

Beef Burgers

Servings|2   Time|25 minutes
Nutritional Content (per serving):
Cal| 212   Fat| 7g   Protein| 34.3g   Carbs| 0.6g   Fiber| 0.1g

Ingredients:

- Lean ground beef (225 grams)
- Fresh coriander (5 grams, minced)
- Pinch of salt
- Garlic clove (1, minced)
- Ground black pepper, as required

Directions:

1. In a bowl, add ground beef, garlic, coriander, salt, and black pepper and with your clean hands, mix well.
2. Make 2 (4-inch) patties from the mixture.
3. Set the temperature of Air Fryer to 195 degrees C to preheat for 5 minutes.
4. After preheating, arrange the patties into the greased Air Fryer Basket in a single layer.
5. Slide the basket into Air Fryer and set the time for 10-11 minutes.
6. After cooking time is finished, remove the patties from Air Fryer and serve hot.

Parsley Pork Loin

Servings|6   Time|35 minutes
Nutritional Content (per serving):
Cal| 261   Fat| 15.7g   Protein| 28.9g   Carbs| 1.2g   Fiber| 0g

Ingredients:

- Pork loin (910 grams)
- Fresh parsley (5 grams, chopped)
- Pinch of salt
- Olive oil (30 milliliters)
- Ground black pepper, as required

Directions:

1. Coat the pork loin with oil and then rub with parsley, salt, and black pepper.
2. Set the temperature of Air Fryer to 165 degrees C to preheat for 5 minutes.
3. After preheating, place the pork loin into the greased Air Fryer Basket.
4. Slide the basket into Air Fryer and set the time for 25 minutes.
5. After cooking time is finished, remove the pork loin from Air Fryer and place onto a platter for about 10 minutes before slicing.
6. Cut the pork loin into desired-sized slices and serve.

Simple Salmon

Servings|2   Time|10 minutes
Nutritional Content (per serving):
Cal| 259   Fat| 16g   Protein| 29.1g   Carbs| 0g   Fiber| 0g

Ingredients:

- ❖ Salmon fillets (2 (150-grams))
- ❖ Ground black pepper, as required
- ❖ Pinch of salt
- ❖ Olive oil (15 milliliters)

Directions:

1. Set the temperature of Air Fryer to 185 degrees C to preheat for 5 minutes.
2. Season each salmon fillet with salt and black pepper and then coat with the oil.
3. After preheating, arrange the salmon fillets into the greased Air Fryer Basket in a single layer.
4. Slide the basket into Air Fryer and set the time for 8-10 minutes.
5. After cooking time is finished, remove the fillets from Air Fryer and serve hot.

Pesto Haddock

Servings|3   Time|20 minutes
Nutritional Content (per serving):
Cal| 351   Fat| 28g   Protein| 26.4g   Carbs| 1.4g   Fiber| 0.4g

Ingredients:

- Haddock fillets (3 (150-grams))
- Pinch of salt
- Pine nuts (30 grams)
- Fresh basil (5 grams, chopped)
- Extra-virgin olive oil (60 milliliters)
- Olive oil (15 milliliters)
- Ground black pepper, as required
- Low-fat Parmesan cheese (15 grams, grated)

Directions:

1. Set the temperature of Air Fryer to 180 degrees C to preheat for 5 minutes.
2. Coat the fish fillets evenly with 15 milliliters of oil and then sprinkle with salt and black pepper.
3. After preheating, arrange the fish fillets into the greased Air Fryer Basket in a single layer.
4. Slide the basket into Air Fryer and set the time for 8 minutes.
5. Meanwhile, for pesto: add the remaining ingredients in a food processor and pulse until smooth.
6. After cooking time is finished, remove the fillets from Air Fryer and place onto serving plates.
7. Top with the pesto and serve.

Roasted Mixed Nuts

Servings|6   Time|25 minutes
Nutritional Content (per serving):
Cal| 176   Fat| 16.3g   Protein| 5.5g   Carbs| 5.5g   Fiber| 3.6g

Ingredients:

- Pecans (60 grams)
- Almonds (50 grams)
- Stevia packet (1)
- Pinch of cayenne pepper
- Walnuts (50 grams)
- Small egg white (1)
- Ground cinnamon (10 grams)

Directions:

1. Set the temperature of Air Fryer to 160 degrees C to preheat for 5 minutes.
2. In a bowl, add all ingredients and toss to coat well.
3. After preheating, place the nuts into the parchment paper-lined Air Fryer Basket in a single layer.
4. Slide the basket into Air Fryer and set the time for 20 minutes.
5. While cooking, shake the basket once halfway through.
6. After cooking time is finished, remove the nuts from Air Fryer and set aside to cool completely before serving.

Banana Chips

Servings|8   Time|20 minutes
Nutritional Content (per serving):
Cal| 57   Fat| 3.7g   Protein| 0.3g   Carbs| 6.7g   Fiber| 0.8g

Ingredients:

- ❖ 2 raw bananas, peeled and sliced
- ❖ Pinch of salt
- ❖ Olive oil (30 milliliters)
- ❖ Ground black pepper, as required

Directions:

1. Set the temperature of Air Fryer to 180 degrees C to preheat for 5 minutes.
2. Drizzle the banana slices with oil evenly.
3. After preheating, arrange the banana slices into the greased Air Fryer Basket in a single layer.
4. Slide the basket into Air Fryer and set the time for 10 minutes.
5. After cooking time is finished, remove the banana chips from Air Fryer and place onto a platter.
6. Sprinkle with salt and black pepper and set aside to cool before serving.

28 Days Meal Plan

Day 1:

Breakfast: Savory Crepes

Lunch: Cucumber & Tomato Salad

Snack: Cheese & Strawberry Bowl

Dinner: Cod with Olives & Tomatoes

Day 2:

Breakfast: Strawberry Chia Pudding

Lunch: Turkey & Beans Lettuce Wraps

Snack: Deviled Eggs

Dinner: Lentil & Quinoa Stew

Day 3:

Breakfast: Beans & Egg Scramble

Lunch: Tuna Sandwich

Snack: Roasted Almonds

Dinner: Steak & Peach Salad

Day 4:

Breakfast: Banana Porridge

Lunch: Spinach Soup

Snack: Quinoa Crackers

Dinner: Parmesan Chicken Bake

Day 5:

Breakfast: Oat & Cheese Waffles

Lunch: Chicken Burgers

Snack: Brinjal Caviar

Dinner: Pork Chops in Sauce

Day 6:

Breakfast: Chicken & Sweet Potato Hash

Lunch: Beef Burgers

Snack: Carrot Sticks

Dinner: Beans & Sweet Potato Chili

Day 7:

Breakfast: Apple Porridge

Lunch: Tuna Sandwich

Snack: Banana Chips

Dinner: Beef & Pumpkin Stew

Day 8:

Breakfast: Oatmeal Pancakes

Lunch: Turkey & Beans Lettuce Wraps

Snack: Cauliflower Poppers

Dinner: Salmon Soup

Day 9:

Breakfast: Apple Omelet

Lunch: Cauliflower Soup

Snack: Roasted Cashews

Dinner: Spiced Chicken Breasts

Day 10:

Breakfast: Savory Crepes

Lunch: Berries & Spinach Salad

Snack: Black Beans Hummus

Dinner: Simple Filet Mignon

Day 11:

Breakfast: Overnight Oatmeal

Lunch: Lemony Shrimp

Snack: Roasted Almonds

Dinner: Herbed Turkey Breast

Day 12:

Breakfast: Spinach & Eggs Bake

Lunch: Salmon Burgers

Snack: Roasted Cashews

Dinner: Lentil & Quinoa Stew

Day 13:

Breakfast: Apple Porridge

Lunch: Spinach Soup

Snack: Berries Gazpacho

Dinner: Steak & Peach Salad

Day 14:

Breakfast: Beans & Egg Scramble

Lunch: Beef Meatballs

Snack: Sweet Potato Croquettes

Dinner: Beans & Sweet Potato Chili

Day 15:

Breakfast: Green Veggies Quiche

Lunch: Chicken & Broccoli Kabobs

Snack: Blueberry Bites

Dinner: Chickpeas & Pumpkin Curry

Day 16:

Breakfast: Savory Crepes

Lunch: Quinoa Lettuce Wraps

Snack: Banana Chips

Dinner: Parsley Pork Loin

Day 17:

Breakfast: Oatmeal Pancakes

Lunch: Stuffed Courgette

Snack: Fish Sticks

Dinner: Ground Turkey Chili

Day 18:

Breakfast: Yogurt & Cheese Bowl

Lunch: Tuna Sandwich

Snack: Sweet Potato Croquettes

Dinner: Chickpeas & Pumpkin Curry

Day 19:

Breakfast: Oat & Cheese Waffles

Lunch: Cauliflower Soup

Snack: Almond Scones

Dinner: Pork Chops in Sauce

Day 20:

Breakfast: Mushroom & Tomato Frittata

Lunch: Beef Meatballs

Snack: carrot Sticks

Dinner: Quinoa & Mango Salad

Day 21:

Breakfast: Chicken & Sweet Potato Hash

Lunch: Berries & Spinach Salad

Snack: Deviled Eggs

Dinner: Parsley Pork Loin

Day 22:

Breakfast: Blueberry Muffins

Lunch: Beef Meatballs

Snack: Cauliflower Poppers

Dinner: Salmon Soup

Day 23:

Breakfast: Apple Omelet

Lunch: Cucumber & Tomato Salad

Snack: Roasted Mixed Nuts

Dinner: Ground Turkey Chili

Day 24:

Breakfast: Pumpkin & Yogurt Bread

Lunch: Lemony Shrimp

Snack: Blueberry Bites

Dinner: Glazed Chicken Drumsticks

Day 25:

Breakfast: Strawberry Chia Pudding

Lunch: Salmon Burgers

Snack: Berries Gazpacho

Dinner: Beef with Cauliflower

Day 26:

Breakfast: Courgette Frittata

Lunch: Chicken & Broccoli Kabobs

Snack: Cheese & Strawberry Bowl

Dinner: Simple Salmon

Day 27:

Breakfast: Overnight Oatmeal

Lunch: Stuffed Courgette

Snack: Quinoa Crackers

Dinner: Shrimp & Tomato Bake

Day 28:

Breakfast: Yogurt & Cheese Bowl

Lunch: Avocado Sandwich

Snack: Fish Sticks

Dinner: Parmesan Chicken Bake

Index

Printed in Great Britain
by Amazon